# Infectious Diseases and Microbiology

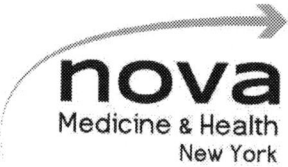

# Infectious Diseases and Microbiology

**Psychological Consequences of the COVID-19 Pandemic on Children, Teenagers and Adults**
Jean-Pascal Assailly, PhD
2022. ISBN: 978-1-68507-963-5 (Softcover)
2022. ISBN: 979-8-88697-072-2 (eBook)

**A Closer Look at the COVID-19 Variants**
Richard D. Hylton (Editor)
2022 ISBN: 979-8-88697-170-5 (Hardcover)
2022 ISBN: 979-8-88697-221-4 (eBook)

**COVID-19: Vaccines, Testing and Compensation Programs**
Mark N. Frierson (Editor)
2022 ISBN: 979-8-88697-167-5 (Hardcover)
2022 ISBN: 979-8-88697-220-7 (eBook)

**Racial Inequities Exposed by COVID-19**
Jamie Isaacson (Editor)
2022 ISBN: 979-8-88697-153-8 (Hardcover)
2022 ISBN: 979-8-88697-188-0 (eBook)

**COVID-19 Vaccines: Development, Distribution and Mandates**
John Schroder (Editor)
2022 ISBN: 979-8-88697-150-7 (Hardcover)
2022 ISBN: 979-8-88697-186-6 (eBook)

More information about this series can be found at
https://novapublishers.com/product-category/series/infectious-diseases-and-microbiology/

Jayapradha Ramakrishnan
and Ganesh Babu Malli Mohan
Editors

# Interdisciplinary Approaches on Opportunistic Infections and Future Prospects

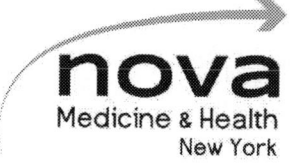

**Copyright © 2022 by Nova Science Publishers, Inc.**
DOI: 10.52305/YBIQ8875.

**All rights reserved.** No part of this book may be reproduced, stored in a retrieval system or transmitted in any form or by any means: electronic, electrostatic, magnetic, tape, mechanical photocopying, recording or otherwise without the written permission of the Publisher.

We have partnered with Copyright Clearance Center to make it easy for you to obtain permissions to reuse content from this publication. Simply navigate to this publication's page on Nova's website and locate the "Get Permission" button below the title description. This button is linked directly to the title's permission page on copyright.com. Alternatively, you can visit copyright.com and search by title, ISBN, or ISSN.

For further questions about using the service on copyright.com, please contact:
Copyright Clearance Center
Phone: +1-(978) 750-8400  Fax: +1-(978) 750-4470  E-mail: info@copyright.com.

## NOTICE TO THE READER

The Publisher has taken reasonable care in the preparation of this book, but makes no expressed or implied warranty of any kind and assumes no responsibility for any errors or omissions. No liability is assumed for incidental or consequential damages in connection with or arising out of information contained in this book. The Publisher shall not be liable for any special, consequential, or exemplary damages resulting, in whole or in part, from the readers' use of, or reliance upon, this material. Any parts of this book based on government reports are so indicated and copyright is claimed for those parts to the extent applicable to compilations of such works.

Independent verification should be sought for any data, advice or recommendations contained in this book. In addition, no responsibility is assumed by the Publisher for any injury and/or damage to persons or property arising from any methods, products, instructions, ideas or otherwise contained in this publication.

This publication is designed to provide accurate and authoritative information with regard to the subject matter covered herein. It is sold with the clear understanding that the Publisher is not engaged in rendering legal or any other professional services. If legal or any other expert assistance is required, the services of a competent person should be sought. FROM A DECLARATION OF PARTICIPANTS JOINTLY ADOPTED BY A COMMITTEE OF THE AMERICAN BAR ASSOCIATION AND A COMMITTEE OF PUBLISHERS.

Additional color graphics may be available in the e-book version of this book.

## Library of Congress Cataloging-in-Publication Data

ISBN: 978-1-68507-984-0

*Published by Nova Science Publishers, Inc. † New York*

# Contents

| | | |
|---|---|---:|
| **Preface** | | vii |
| **Chapter 1** | **Interdisciplinary Studies on Opportunistic Fungal Pathogens and Their Future Perspectives** | 1 |
| | Jananishree Sathiyamoorthy, Murugavel Aravind and Jayapradha Ramakrishnan | |
| **Chapter 2** | **Interdisciplinary Mathematical Modeling Approaches for Infectious Diseases** | 41 |
| | Gottumukkala Sai Bhavani, Sumathi Kalankariyan, Lavanya Sargunam and Anbumathi Palanisamy | |
| **Chapter 3** | **Immunomodulation and Immunotherapy to Tackle Opportunistic Infections** | 71 |
| | Sayed Muhammad Ata Ullah Shah Bukhari, Liloma Shah, Sana Raza and Muhsin Jamal | |
| **Chapter 4** | **Genetically Engineered Bacteriophages for the Treatment of ESKAPE Pathogens** | 105 |
| | Haseesh Rahithya Nandam, Anjali Parmar, Krithikashri Sarathy and Sutharsan Govindarajan | |
| **Chapter 5** | **Pathogenesis of Opportunistic Infections** | 123 |
| | Salini Krishnarao Kandhalu and K. V. Murali Mohan | |
| **Editors' Contact Information** | | 151 |
| **Index** | | 153 |

# Preface

The improvement in medical advances incidentally has led to an increase in the incidence of opportunistic infections (OIs) in immune-compromised patients. The OIs are the major cause of severity in illness and death in HIV, cancer patients, tuberculosis, organ transplant recipients, malnutrition, preterm babies etc. OIs are a growing concern as the microbe takes advantage when the immune system is weak. Even the microbes that reside in us for many years may cause serious disease when the immune system has weakened. Also, certain microbes get reactivated and cause opportunistic infections. Such common OIs include oral and pharyngeal candidiasis, tuberculosis, herpes zoster, bacterial pneumonia, cryptococcal meningitis, and toxoplasmosis. Such secondary infections are common in immunocompromised and long-term hospitalized severely ill patients. Currently, the incidence of secondary infections is increased world-wide in COVID-19 infected patients. Treating opportunistic infections in COVID-19, AIDS and various other immune compromised patients is a nightmare when they are already under heavy drug dosage and immunity loss. In addition, antimicrobial resistance is a serious hazard and prolonged medication for fungal infections in immune-compromised patients can lead to adverse effects such as nephrotoxicity. The increased rate of antimicrobial resistance in bacteria, causing treatment failure, warrants much attention worldwide. There is extreme need of innovative and novel approaches. Also, the tracking of epidemics/pandemics, their dynamics and patterns are required as an important controlling strategy. Understanding the molecular mechanism of host pathogen interactions facilitates the discoveries of new drug targets. Alternative approaches like immune modulation and phage therapy hold numerous advantages over antibiotic therapy including targeting of a specific pathogen. This book, we believe, will serve as a small but important piece of source material for students and researchers interested in this particular area of research. The chapters are divided to showcase the relevance and importance of interdisciplinary approaches to tackle infectious diseases such as mathematical modeling, omics, immunomodulation, immunotherapy, and genetic engineering of bacteriophages for phage therapy. We hope that the topics will kindle the interest of young researchers. In the end, we are grateful and wholeheartedly acknowledge the authors for their valuable contribution and reviewers for their valuable suggestions and critical review of the chapters. The editors sincerely thank the funding agency, Science & Research Engineering Board, Department of Science & Technology, Government of India and SASTRA Deemed to be University, India.

*Dr. Jayapradha Ramakrishnan*
Associate Professor
Centre for Research in Infectious Diseases
SASTRA (Deemed to be University), India

*Dr. Ganesh Babu Malli Mohan*
Assistant Professor
Centre for Research in Infectious Diseases
SASTRA (Deemed to be University), India

Chapter 1

# Interdisciplinary Studies on Opportunistic Fungal Pathogens and Their Future Perspectives

## Jananishree Sathiyamoorthy[1], Murugavel Aravind[2] and Jayapradha Ramakrishnan[*]

Actinomycetes Bioprospecting Lab,
Centre for Research in Infectious Diseases (CRID),
School of Chemical and Biotechnology,
SASTRA (Deemed to be University),
Thanjavur, Tamil Nadu, India

## Abstract

The phenomenon of opportunistic fungal infections has increased in recent decades because of the expansion of at-risk populations as an outcome of immunosuppression. Corresponding to several environmentally seized fungal diseases, *Cryptococcus* spp., *Mucor* spp., and *Rhizopus* spp. commences infection in the lungs and then gets disseminated. Such fungal infections cause indicative morbidity and mortality because they tend to breach blood vessels and infect vital organs. There are several emerging high-risk opportunistic angioinvasive fungal diseases worldwide. This chapter focuses on Mucormycosis and Cryptococcosis. The chapter deals with their interdisciplinary aspects, including emergence, virulence, evolution, epidemiology, omics tools, host defense, diagnostics, and treatment strategies.

---

[*] Corresponding Author's Email: antibioticbiology@gmail.com.

In: Interdisciplinary Approaches on Opportunistic Infections ...
Editors: Jayapradha Ramakrishnan and Ganesh Babu Malli Mohan
ISBN: 978-1-68507-984-0
© 2022 Nova Science Publishers, Inc.

# 1. Mucormycosis

## 1.1. Introduction

Mucormycosis is an infrequent but serious life-threatening angioinvasive fungal infection, previously called zygomycosis (Skiada et al., 2011, Prakash et al., 2021). Mucormycosis usually affects an immunocompromised person, which means the pathogen acts opportunistically (Hernández et al., 2019). Mucormycosis is not a communicable disease, which means it doesn't transmit between humans or between animals and humans (Kouadio et al., 2012). Mucormycosis is caused by a group of ubiquitous saprophytic filamentous fungi associated with the class Zygomycetes (Hoffmann et al., 2013). All Mucormycosis causing fungus belongs to the sub-phylum Mucormycotina, whereas some are recently classified into the sub-phylum Entomophthoramycotina. Most of the Mucormycosis-causing pathogens belong to the order Mucorales (Ribes et al., 2000 and Spellberg et al., 2005). The fungi belonging to Mucorales emerge as large, aseptate, or sparsely septate with ribbon-like hyphae. It includes nearly 11 genera and approximately 27 species that are associated with human infections (Jeong et al., 2019). These fungi commonly exist everywhere in the environment. They mostly live in decaying organic matter such as leaves, compost piles, or rotten wood in the soil. They are predominant in summer and fall rather than in winter or spring. The comprehensive mortality rate for Mucormycosis persists at ~50% and it approaches over 90% in patients with disseminated disease or those with persistent neutropenia (Ibrahim et al., 2012). The estimated ubiquity of Mucormycosis is approximately 70 times more elevated than the global data (Prakash et al., 2021). Generally, Mucormycosis involve vital organs such as the nose, sinus, CNS, lungs, GI tract, skin, jawbones, joints, heart, kidney, and mediastinum (Singh et al., 2021).

## 1.2. Causative Agents

The common fungal species that serve as a source of Mucormycosis are *Rhizopus* spp., (especially *Rhizopus oryzae*), and *Mucor* spp. Other species encompasses *Rhizomucor* spp., *Syncephalastrum* spp., *Cunninghamellaber-tholletiae*, *Apophysomyces* spp., *Lichtheimiacorymbifera* (formerly *Absidia*), *Saksenaea*, and *Rhizomucor* (Neblett et al., 2012).

Among all the causative agents, *Rhizopus delemar* (formerly called *Rhizopus oryzae*) and *Mucor circinelloides* are the most commonly isolated organisms from approximately 70% of Mucormycosis patients (Gracia et al., 2018). In India, *Rhizopus arrhizus* is the preeminent cause of Mucormycosis, but illnesses due to *Rhizopus microspores*, *Rhizopus homothallicus*, and *Apophysomyces* variabilis are rising. Occasionally, *Sakenaeaerythrospora*, *Mucor irregularis*, and *Thamnostylumlucknowense* were also isolated (Borkar2021).

## 1.3. Types of Mucormycosis

The major clinical forms of Mucormycosis based on anatomical localization include:

### *1.3.1. Rhino Orbital Cerebral Mucormycosis (ROCM)*
It is a condition affecting the sinuses that can proliferate to the brain. It is almost common for people with unbound diabetes. Additionally, it can occur in neutropenic cancer patients and transplant recipients who have received hematopoietic stem cells or solid organ transplants (Gamaletsou et al., 2012). Trauma is one of the risk factors of ROCM, mainly after contaminated dental procedures during tooth extraction.

### *1.3.2. Pulmonary Mucormycosis*
People suffering from hematologic malignancy and people who have undergone an organ or a stem cell transplant are commonly susceptible to pulmonary Mucormycosis. It also affects patients suffering from profound neutropenia, kidney malfunction, and hematologic cancers (Lee et al., 1999).

### *1.3.3. Gastrointestinal Mucormycosis (GIMucormycosis)*
It is rarer than the other forms and it results from ingestion of the organism. It is highly prevalent among neonates. Infants born prematurely or with low birth weight will have an increased risk of infection if they have been treated with antibiotics, undergone surgery, or taken a medication that lowers the immune system. Neutropenic adults are also at risk (Spellberg and Brad 2012). Malnourished patients are also susceptible to GI Mucormycosis. It mostly affects the stomach, colon, and ileum. The challenging part is diagnosis

because the disease is clinically similar to necrotizing enterocolitis, a much more common disorder.

### 1.3.4. Cutaneous (Skin) Mucormycosis:
### It Is the Third Most Recurrent Form of Mucormycosis

Skin Mucormycosisoccurs after the fungal entry into the body through the disrupted skin. This might occur after a burn, scrape, cut, surgery, or other types of skin trauma (Skiada et al., 2013). This is the most common form of Mucormycosis among immunocompetent people.

### 1.3.5. Disseminated Mucormycosis

It occurs once the infection proliferates through the bloodstream to infect vital organs of the body. The infection most commonly affects the brain but also can affect other organs such as the spleen, heart, and skin. It is typically observed in neutropenic patients with a lung infection, patients who have undergone transplant surgery, or patients undergoing deferoxamine therapy (Sarrami et al, 2013).

## 1.4. Transmission

The primary route of transmission is the inhalation of fungal spores. Infectious propagules are often spread by way of the nasal cavity, which is considered to be the major pathway to the lungs. The dissemination of fungal spores in immunocompromised patients is shown in Figures 1a and 1b.

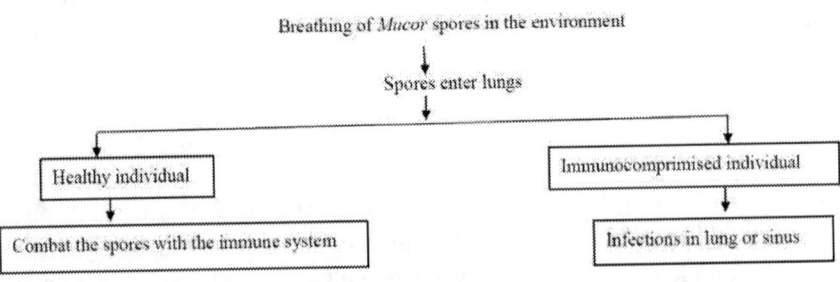

**Figure 1a.** Transmission of Mucormycosis.

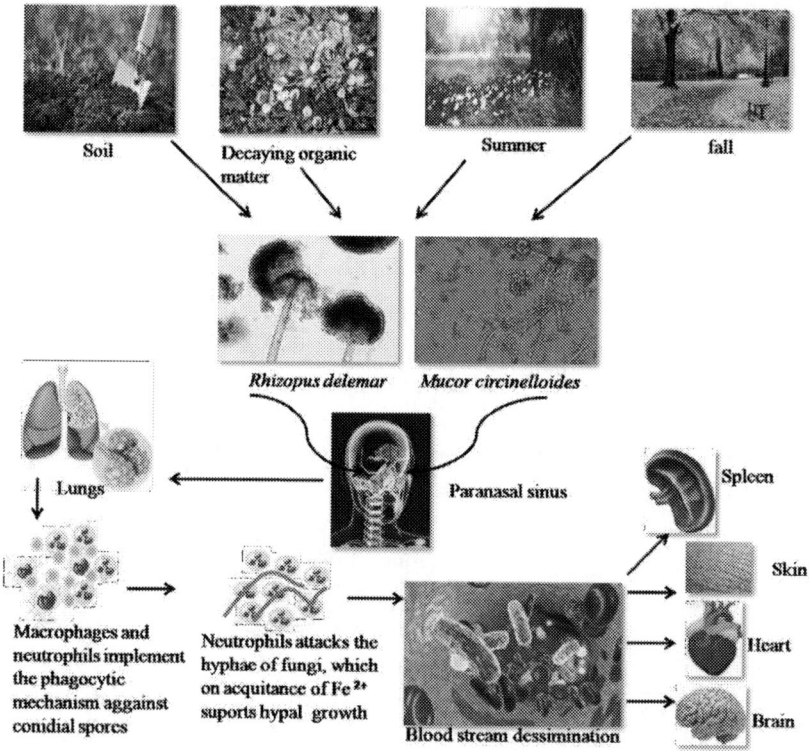

**Figure 1b.** Pathogenesis of Mucormycosis.

## 1.5. Host Defense Mechanisms

Mucoralean fungi could break through the epithelial cells of the host which is the first line of defense and it was recently found that the intensification of the infection is increased due to the overexpression of Platelet-Derived Growth Factor Receptor B (PDGFRB). Individuals who lack phagocyte cells or who have lower phagocyte count are at augmented risk of developing Mucormycosis infection. Hence sufferers of severe neutropenia are more susceptible than AIDS patients (Suganya et al., 2019). Both mononuclear and polymorphonuclear phagocytes kill the Mucorales by secreting oxidative metabolites, cationic peptides, and defensins (Waldorf et al., 1984, Waldorf and Alayn 1989, Diamond et al., 1982). As a result of exposure to *R.delemar*hyphae, neutrophils exhibit TLR-2 (Toll-like receptors) overexpression as well as robust proinflammatory gene expression (IL-1B), with rapid activation of nuclear factor kappa-B(NF-κB) pathway-related genes. (Chamilos et al., 2008). TNF-α released from neutrophils leads to hyphal damage and helps in eradicating Mucormycosis. In patients with diabetic ketoacidosis (DKA) (hyperglycemia and low pH) phagocytes are defective and have flawed chemotaxis and dysfunctional intracellular killing by both oxidative and nonoxidative mechanisms (Chinn and Richard 1982).

Accordant with these clinical observations, inhaling Mucorales sporangio spores by an immunocompetent individual has no effect on the person for developing Mucormycosis (Waldorf et al., 1984). Distinct immunosuppressed persons especially with DKA have more chances of mortality due to progressive pulmonary and hematogenously disseminated infection. The pulmonary alveolar macrophages can ingest and inhibit the germination of morale sporangiospores, whereas the bronchoalveolar macrophages have only defined capacity to decimate the organism in vitro. The mechanism by which the phagocytes become dysfunctional by ketoacidosis, Diabetes mellitus, and corticosteroids is yet to be resolved. Mucorales influence distinctive virulence traits that enable the organism to utilize the unique state of immunosuppression and physiologic impairment seen in patients (Ibrahim and Spellberg 2012). The skin acts as a physical barrier against cutaneous Mucormycosis, as evidenced by the developing Mucormycosis in persons with disruption in the barrier. The Mucormycosis pathogens are capable of penetrating intact skin. However, the patients with disrupted skin due to burns, traumatic disruption, and persistent maceration of skin enable the organism to penetrate deeper tissues. It is believed to have arisen from the traumatic implantation of contaminated soil or water.

In addition, contaminated surgical equipment and dressings, and nonsterile adhesive tapes are responsible for cutaneous Mucormycosis. Furthermore, Mucormycosis can even seep through contaminated tongue depressors of neonates or the contaminated wooden applicators used to mix drugs given to immunocompromised patients. Mucormycosis is both a community-acquired and nosocomial infection (Ibrahim et. al., 2012).

**1.6. Mucormycosis Pathogenesis: Mucorales Hold Certain Virulence Factors That Let the Organism Survive the Disease By Bypassing the Host's Defense Mechanisms**

*1.6.1. Iron Uptake*
The first virulence trait is the organism's potential to attain iron from the host. Iron plays a crucial role in human cell growth and development, contributing

to many important processes within the cell (Howard and Dexter 1999). Hence a successful pathogen utilizes numerous processes for acquiring iron from the host. The level of free, unbound iron in the serum plays a condemnatory factor in uniquely predisposing patients with DKA to Mucormycosis (Artis et al., 1982, Boelaert et al., 1993). In mammals, the iron is bounded by a carrier protein transferrin, ferritin, or lactoferrin. Such sequestration helps to circumvent the toxic effects of free iron (Howard and Dexter 1999, Boelaert et al., 1993). Over a while, the free iron accumulates in the internal organs, causing potentially fatal damage to the brain and liver. The free iron also results in the generation of Reactive Oxygen Species (ROS) (Eid et al., 2017). The strategy of iron-binding to a carrier protein is also defined to be an important host defense mechanism against various pathogens including Mucorales in particular *R. delemar* grows poorly in normal serum (Artis et al., 1982). The iron uptake in Rhizopus spp. takes place in three different mechanisms. The first mechanism embraces Reductive Iron Assimilation (RIA) is an uninterrupted process that involves 3 major enzymes, which is been used to obtain iron from the host (Ibrahim et al., 2012).

**Table 1.** Genes and their function taking part in Iron acquisition (Lax et al., 2020)

| S.no. | Gene involved | Name of the enzyme | The function of the enzyme |
|---|---|---|---|
| 1. | FRE5 | Ferric reductase | Reduces the iron (Stanford et al., 2020) |
| 2. | FET3 | Multicopper ferroxidase | Reoxidation of iron (Stanford et al., 2020) |
| 3. | FTR1 | High-affinity Iron permease | Translocation across membrane (Ibrahim et al., 2012) |

The second mechanism involves the potential of fungi to synthesize and or exploit low molecular weight siderophores are iron chelators (Howard and Dexter 1999). The final mechanism engages heme oxygenase to release iron from heme. The genes and enzymes involved in these processes are considered to be the virulence determinants for fungal pathogens as iron metabolism plays a central role in the development of Mucormycosis. Rhizopus spp. has the potential to exude rhizoferrin that dispenses Rhizopus spp. with iron which is an energy-dependent process (Thieken et al., 1992).

Patients with diabetic ketoacidosis are uniquely prone to Mucormycosis because of raised levels of free iron in the serum, which supports the growth of *R. delemar* at pH 7.78-8.83 (Spellberg et al., 2005). Acidic conditions in the blood disrupt the iron uptake of Mucorales by siderophores (Spellberg et al., 2005). Iron chelators also help to protect the patient from predisposing Mucormycosis (Binder et al., 2013). Fungi use mechanisms like high-affinity iron permeases or low-molecular-weight iron chelators (siderophores) to procure iron from the host. The contagious cells (fungal cells) have high-affinity iron permeases as a portion of the reductive framework containing dispensable surface reductase that decreases ferric form to a more soluble ferrous form. The diminished ferrous form created by the surface reductase is in turn, seized by a protein complex that comprises a multicopper oxidase and a ferrous permease (Jung et al., 2008, Ibrahim et al., 2012). The high- affinity iron permease is considered a crucial virulence factor.

### *1.6.2. Genes Promoting Drug Resistance in Mucor Circinelloides*

In *Mucor circinelloides*, the Pleiotropic drug resistance (PDR) family of genes promotes resistance to the class of azole drugs by the mechanism of azole efflux. The PDR family is a cluster of genes composed of *PDR1, PDR2, PDR3, PDR4, PDR5, PDR6, PDR7, PDR8*, and *AFR1* (Nagetal., 2021). All PDR genes are highly interconnected and correlated. *pdr1* and *pdr2* play a vital role in protecting the pathogen from the consequence of posaconazole, isavuconazole, and ravuconazole (Nagy et al., 2021). *PDR1* alone provides resistance against posaconazole, isavuconazole. The function of the *PDR1* gene is affected by oxygen levels in the environment. The next class of genes is Calcineurin genes that take part in the dimorphic transition of Mucor. *AFR1* gene shows resistance to fluconazole and is also responsible for increasing the virulence of the Mucorales (Chang et al., 2018). PKAR set of genes helps in the viability of fungal cells and dimorphic transition. *CnbR* gene is a calcineurin regulatory subunit that plays a role in calcium binding and calcium-dependent protein serine/threonine phosphatase. Cna A gene helps in the hyphal growth of *Mucor*. *Cnb R* and *Cna A* genes induce larger- sized spores. CotHgene codes for spore coat proteins that perpetrate virulence mechanisms. *PYRG* and *LEUA* genes serve as auxotrophic markers (Gracia et. al., 2018). *CAR* gene helps in carotene production.

### 1.7. Mucorales and the World of Omics

Though there is much evidence for the molecular mechanisms, genome structure, etc., for pathogenic fungi like Aspergillus spp., Candida spp., and

Saccharomyces spp., the evidence of molecular mechanisms for Mucorales is not well known. The reason behind the knowledge gap in such a large part between other pathogenic fungi and Mucorales is the intractable nature of the genome of Mucorales. It is evident that there is a large evolutionary distance between Mucorales from Ascomycetes and Basidiomycetes. Certain strategies used to study the genome of Mucorales include gene deletion and RNAi-based knockdown studies that provide valuable insights into the molecular pathogenic mechanism of Mucormycosis. But still, the availability of omics data in this particular pathogen is low (Ibrahim et al., 2010, Gracia et al., 2018). Next-generation sequencing technologies provide important insights and investigational avenues for better understanding, diagnosing, and developing alarmingly needed therapies for such emerging diseases.

R. delemar is identified with a highly repetitive genome structure, which is an indication of ancestral whole-genome duplication (WGD) event. The WGD occasion comes about within the replication of gene families related to cell development, flag transduction, and cell divider amalgamation (Ma et al., 2009). Mucoromycotina subdivision of fungi has the highest gene duplication. The genome sequences of Rhizopus spp. have an exceptional variety of genome lengths. There's an enhancement within the structure of the mating-type locus inside the Rhizopus genome that contrasts with the classic course of action of Mucoromycotina (Gryganskyi et al., 2018). It is also found that most of the Mucorales have the highest number of transposable elements (Prakash et al., 2017).

### 1.7.1. ChIP (Chromatin Immunoprecipitation)
ChIP (Chromatin immunoprecipitation) of *M. circinelloides* stated a unique "mosaic" centromere in Mucoromycotina which is a characteristic difference between point centromere and regional centromeres (Navarro- Mendoza et al., 2019).

### 1.7.2. RNA Sequencing
RNA sequencing provides a wide knowledge of germination and hyphal growth of the Mucorales. Transcriptomic analysis was performed in a time-dependent fashion. *R. delemerspores* have distinct gene clusters. The gene expression in *R. delemarhappens* in a time-dependent design in understanding with formative stages of parasitic growth. Most of the transcriptional changes occurred within the first hour of germination then there is a transcriptional consistency during isotropic swelling. During the transition from dormant to hyphal growth, there is a switchover in gene expression. In the dormant spore

stage, there is an increased expression of lipid storage genes and localization genes. These genes provide energy to the Mucorales during the starvation period. In *R. delemar* fatty acid metabolism is involved amongst differentially regulated genes during the change from mycelia form to pellet-like morphology (Xu Q. et al., 2018). The transcriptomic analyses of Mucorales provide evidence of lipid metabolism which gives the ability to Mucorales to utilize Trehalose as a carbon source and produce gamma-linolenic acid. The change in lipid metabolism takes place when there is a long-term high-temperature change occurred (Soare et al., 2020).

A few genes are upregulated which makes a difference to outlive a hypoxic environment. *R. delemar* produces twofold the number of chitin synthase and chitin deacetylase. In reaction to oxidative push, *R. delemar* upregulates qualities related to chitin catabolism, most likely to reduce the chitin composition within the cell divider and diminish ROS harm. Genes included in cell divider biosynthesis and compositions are differentially communicated as *R. delemar* experiences germination. There's still a part of certainty to be divulged in ergosterol biosynthesis (Soare et al., 2020).

One of the major classes of virulence genes is *CotH*proteins which is the major class of spore coat proteins. Nearly six to seven copies of *CotH*genes were isolated from the strains collected from infected patients. Among the various *CotH*proteins *CotH3*, *CotH2* and *CotH8* are highly expressed. *CotH3* is considered to be the most virulent protein. The Mucorales which do not cause disease in humans lack these homologs *CotH*genes. This establishes that the number of *CotH*genes in the genome is proportional to its potential to invade and cause impairment in the host cell. The next class of virulence factors is the secreted proteases which are majorly present in *R. delemar* (Chibucos et al., 2016). It has many gene families of proteases. The secondary metabolites are produced by upregulation of certain genes that secrete a toxin which results in causing food-borne illness. Both pathogenic and non-pathogenic Mucorales have the same set of secondary metabolites production. The third major class of virulence promotion is iron acquisition.

*R. delemer* needs non-ribosomal peptide synthetases that deliver common siderophores. But it encodes Rhizoferrin a siderophore with two duplicates of quality encoding heme oxygenase. Amid pathogenesis *FET3* a multicopper ferroxidase capable of ferrous press take-up and parasitic dimorphism is communicated in a raised amount. *FTR1* is a tall partiality permease that is profoundly communicated amid contagious dimorphism. Amid thetorpid arrange there's an upregulation of press procurement qualities. RNAi silencing does not affect the gene expression of growth, acidic pH, and sexual interaction. RNAi silencing suggests that these processes are regulated by a dicer independent non-canonical pathway (NCRIP) which plays a considerable role in controlling the harmfulness of Mucorales (Pérez-Arques et al., 2020). The functional role of NCRIP includes the regulation of mRNA expression, maintaining the genome stability by regulating the expression of retrotransposon, and regulation of response during phagocytosis that affects the multifaceted process of virulence (Cánovas-Márquez et al., 2021). Novel RNAi machinery is present in *Mucor circinelloides* which provides antifungal resistance elucidated through RNA sequencing on small RNAs. Antimicrobial resistance genes of Mucorales are *fbA*, *pyrF*, and *pyrG*. In *R. delemar* and *M. circinelloides*, certain enrichment genes act against platelet-derived growth factor receptor beta (PDGFRB) and epidermal growth factor receptor (EFGR) of the host (Soare et al., 2020).

## 1.8. Susceptible Community

Certain groups of individuals are more likely to urge Mucormycosis, counting individuals with uncontrolled diabetes, particularly with diabetic ketoacidosis, metabolic acidosis, cancer, solid organ transplant, Drunkard, stem cell transplant, bone marrow transplant, injury post pneumonic tuberculosis, persistent obstructive aspiratory infection, asthma persistent kidney infections, neutropenia (moo number of white blood cells), long-term corticosteroid utilize (Steroid treatment), deferoxamine treatment, infusion drug use, tall press collection within the body (press over-burden or hemochromatosis), dangerous hematologic disarranges, inveterate liquor abuse, skin damage due to surgery, burns, or wounds, rashness and lower birthweight (for neonatal gastrointestinal Mucormycosis) (Gracia et al., 2018 and Ghuman and Voelz, 2017).

## 1.9. Epidemiology of Mucormycosis

### *1.9.1. India*
Rhino orbital cerebral Mucormycosis is considered to be the most common type of Mucormycosis in India. Isolated renal Mucormycosis is considered to be a unique clinical presentation in India (Zaman et al., 2017). The intracranial involvement of Mucormycosis increased the chances of fatality to 90% (Prakash et al., 2021).

In Southern India (especially in Tamil Nadu) two epidemiological study was made for a period of 10 years (From 2005- to 2015) (Manesh et al., 2019) and 5 years (From 2015- to 2019) (Priya et al., 2020). On contrastive analysis, the incidence of Mucormycosis is reduced. Among the various risk factors, Diabetes mellitus and DKA are considered to be the top predisposing factors of Mucormycosis in South India (Tamil Nadu) that varying from 17- 88% globally (Prakash et al., 2021). In North India (especially in Chandigarh) two epidemiological study was made for a period of 15 years (From 1990- to 2004) and 5 years (From 2010 to 2014) (Chander et al., 2018). In the first study, it is estimated that around 382 people were affected with Mucoromycosis, and in the second report; it is only around 82 affected people. Comparatively, after 2010, the incidence of Mucormycosis is slightly reduced. Among the various risk factors, the most common are diabetes mellitus and DKA. The other risk factors include solid organ transplant, breach of skin, pulmonary diseases, neutropenia, steroid therapy, chronic alcoholism, chronic kidney diseases, HIV, Immunocompetent host, etc. North India also reported that 12% of Mucormycosis is of nosocomial origin (Prakash et al., 2021). The nosocomial spread may occur due to defile intramuscular injections, surgery, adhesive tapes, and endobronchialtubes.

### *1.9.2. Mucoromysis Chronological Order Based on Its Prevalence*
ROCM (45-74%) > Cutaneous Mucormycosis (10-31%) > Pulmonary Mucormycosis (3-22%) > Renal Mucormycosis (0.5-9%) > Gastrointestinal Mucormycosis (2-8%) > Disseminated Mucormycosis (0.5-9%) (Prakash et al., 2021).

### *1.9.3. Global Epidemiology of Mucormycosis*
Globally the Mucormycosis infection survey was taken and it is perceived that the Asian continent (especially India) (Singh et al., 2021) has the highest infection rate. The major mode of contamination is through the inward breath of sporangiospores, and seldom by ingestion of sullied nourishment or traumatic vaccination. Within the Asian landmass, Diabetes Mellitus is considered the major hazard calculates while in European nations and US, hematological malignancies and transplantation are the major hazard components (Singh et al., 2021). In modern, healthcare-associated (Nosocomial) Mucormycosis is progressively archived. Within the Asian landmass, India and China are considered to be the topmost reoccurring *Mucor* diseases which are due to uncontrolled Diabetes mellitus.

Planned observation among 16,808 transplant beneficiaries performed in 23 institutions from 2001 to 2006 found that Mucormycosis was the third most common sort of obtrusive fungal disease in stem cell transplant beneficiaries and accounted for 8% of all obtrusive invasive fungal diseases. In 983 stem cell transplant beneficiaries 77 Mucoromycete cases were reported (Kontoyiannis et al., 2010). Among solid-organ transplant beneficiaries, Mucormycosis accounted for 2% of all intrusive contagious diseases (Stop et. al., 2011, Pappas et. al., 2010). The number of cases varied broadly over participating institutions.

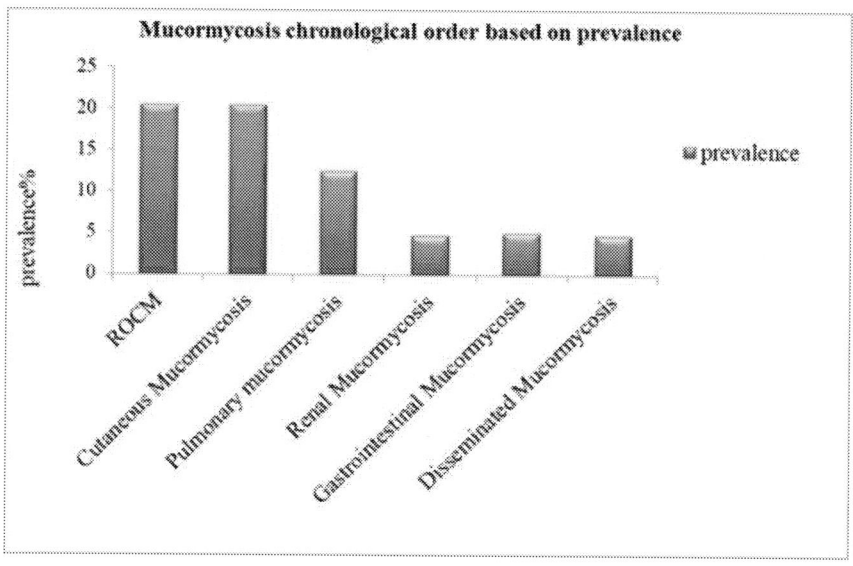

**Figure 2.** Mucormycosis chronological order based on prevalence.

## 1.10. Mucormycosis and COVID-19

Aspergillosis and Candidiasis have been reported as the major fungal infection associated with COVID-19, but the scenario changed when there was an increased case of rhino orbital Mucormycosis in people with COVID-19 worldwide, especially in India (Singh et al., 2021).

The primary causes that paved the way for Mucormycosis infection in people with COVID-19 includes:
- Hypoxia

- High glucose
  - Diabetes induced hyperglycemia
  - Steroid induced hyperglycemia
- DKA
- High iron
- Decreased phagocytic activity
- Prolonged hospital stay with or without ventilators (Singh et al., 2021).

The reoccurrence of Mucormycosis is nearly 80 times higher in India contrasted to developed countries globally in a recent estimate of 2019 to 2020 (Singh et al., 2021). Diabetes mellitus, the leading cause of Mucormycosis globally has resulted in an estimate of 46% of overall mortality (Hoang et al., 2020). According to the European Confederation of Medical Mycology study, 46% of patients who had received corticosteroids are diagnosed with Mucormycosis in a gap of a month. Hence it is concluded that corticosteroid therapy increased the prevalence of Mucormycosis globally.

COVID-19 frequently causes endothelialitis, endothelial damage, thrombosis, lymphopenia, and reduction in CD4 and CD8 T-cell levels and thus predisposes to secondary or opportunistic fungal infection. The high amount of free iron is considered to be the ideal source for Mucormycosis.

## 1.11. Mortality Due to Mucormycosis

Mucormycosis is a life-threatening disease. An audit of Mucormycosis cases found a broad all-cause mortality rate of 54%. The mortality rate is grouped depending on basic persistent condition, sort of organism, and body location influenced (for illustration, the mortality rate was 46% among individuals with sinus contaminations, 76% for aspiratory diseases, and 96% for spread Mucormycosis) (Roden et al., 2005).

## 1.12. Symptoms of Mucormycosis

Giant cell invasion, thrombosis, and eosinophilic necrosis of the underlying tissue are the major hallmarks of Mucormycosis.

**Table 2. Symptoms of Mucormycosis**

|  | Primary symptoms | Secondary symptoms |
|---|---|---|
| ROCM | • Unilateral(One-sided) facial swelling<br>• Headache<br>• Nasal or sinus congestion, or pain<br>• Serosanguinous nasal discharge<br>• Fever (Abdollahi et al., 2016) | • Ptosis<br>• Proptosis<br>• Loss of extraocular muscle function<br>• Vision disturbance may occur<br>• Necrotic black lesions on the hard palate or nasal turbinate and drainage of black pus from the eyes, cranial nerve palsy (Abdollahi et al., 2016). |
| Cutaneous Mucormycosis | • Acute inflammatory response with pus<br>• Abscess formation,<br>• Tissue swelling<br>• Necrosis<br>• The injuries may show up ruddy and indurated and frequently advance to dark eschars. (Pérez et al., 2017). | Injuries regularly start as an erythematous, indurated, and periorbital cellulitis and after that advance to an ulcer secured with a dark eschar (Pérez et al.,2017). |
| Pulmonary Mucormycosis | • Fever<br>• Cough<br>• Chest pain<br>• Dyspnea (Shortness of breath), hypoxia, and<br>• Hemoptysis (Maqeetadnan et al., 2012). | Angioinvasion comes about in tissue corruption, which may eventually lead to cavitation and/or hemoptysis. |
| Gastrointestinal Mucormycosis | • Abdominal pain<br>• Nausea<br>• Vomiting, gastrointestinal bleeding, and distension<br>• Fever | Hematochezia and intra-abdominal abscess might occur (Spellberg and Brad 2012). |

**Table 2.** (Continued)

| | Primary symptoms | Secondary symptoms |
|---|---|---|
| Disseminated Mucormycosis | Disseminated Mucormycosis ordinarily happens in individuals who are as of now wiped out from other restorative conditions, so it can be troublesome to know which indications are related to Mucormycosis. Patients with the dispersed disease within the brain can create mental status changes or coma. | |

## 1.13. Diagnosis

In 1950 Smith and Kirchner standardized the clinical diagnosis of Mucormycosis that is still considered the gold standard and include:

1. Black, necrotic turbinate's easily mistaken for dried, crustedblood
2. Blood-tinged nasal discharge and facial pain, both on the sameside
3. Soft peri-orbital or peri-nasal swelling with discoloration and induration
4. Ptosis of the eyelid, proptosis of the eyeball, and complete ophthalmoplegia
5. Multiple cranial nerve palsies unrelated to documentedlesions

### 1.13.1. Diagnostic Procedures

The determination of Mucormycosis depends on the distinguishing proof of living beings in tissues by histopathology together with cultural affirmation. PCR-based strategies on histopathologic specimens are considered a promising apparatus for building up the conclusion of Mucormycosis (Lackner et al., 2021). MALDI- TOF mass spectrometry can moreover be utilized to recognize the causative species from culture specimens (Schrödl,et al., 2012, Cassagne et al., 2011). Patients with ROCM have changed mental action and infracted tissue within the nose or sense of taste. A nendoscopic assessment of sinuses is to be performed to see the corruption of the tissue and to gather the example. Calcofluor white, methenamine silverstains, Periodic acid Schiff and hematoxylin and eosin staining are utilized to imagine the irresistible organism's morphology, (Lass-Flörl 2009). CT scans are considered the primary imaging due to their affectability and speed. The discoveries of the CT scan incorporate serious delicate soft tissue edema of nasal cavity mucus, sinus mucoperiosteal thickening, bone erosion, orbital invasion, facial soft tissue swelling, and retrolental fatpad (Lass-Flörl 2009). Pulmonary Mucormycosis is difficult to diagnose as it is difficult to differentiate Mucormycosis from pneumonia due to other angioinvasive molds. A definitive diagnosis is difficult as it requires a demonstration of the organism in tissue. Chestradiographs or CT scans may demonstrate focal consolidation, masses, pleural effusions, or multiple nodules. Sputumor- bronchoalveolar lavage (BAL) specimens show the characteristic broad non- septate hyphae, which is often the first indicator of Mucormycosis (Skiadaetal., 2020). Lung biopsy is another diagnostic technique to characterize the hyphae.

The determination of gastrointestinal Mucormycosis can be made with an endoscopic biopsy of the injuries that appear in the characteristic hyphae. Percutaneous biopsy or nephrectomy can build up a determination for renal inclusion. Imaging of the kidneys with a CT scan illustrates either ill-defined ranges of low attenuation and reduced improvement suggestive of pyelonephritis or numerous little foci suggestive of abscesses.

## 1.14. Treatments

### 1.14.1. Antifungal Therapy

Mucormycosis could be genuine contamination and should be treated with medicine antifungal medication, ordinarily amphotericin B, posaconazole, or isavuconazole (Sipsas et al., 2018). These solutions are given intravenous (amphotericin B, posaconazole, isavuconazole) or oral (posaconazole, isavuconazole). Other medications, counting fluconazole, voriconazole, and echinocandins, don't work against parasites that cause Mucormycosis. Often, Mucormycosis requires surgical debridement of contaminated tissue. Since the conclusive determination was troublesome within the case of Mucormycosis, numerous patients will be treated as they have hazard variables for Mucormycosis contamination and positive societies and consistent clinical disorders. Lipid definition of amphotericin B (5 mg/kg day by day) in intravenous mode is the essential sedate of choice (Tissot et al.,

2017). Once the patients begin reacting to the amphotericin B, the next medicine of choice is posaconazole (300 mg once in 12 hours on day 1then 300 mg per day (Sipsas et al., 2018) or isavuconazole which is considered to be the step-down therapy. Patients allergic to amphotericin B are fundamentally treated with posaconazole or isavuconazole and this kind of treatment is called rescue treatment. Posaconazole or isavuconazole can be given either by oral or IV based on the escalated ailment inpatients.

### 1.14.2. Surgery
Forceful surgical debridements of included tissues are considered as and when any frame of Mucormycosis is suspected and analyzed. Evacuation of necrotic tissue and surgical debulking are related to moving forward survival rates. (Tissot et al., 2017, Chowdary et al., 2014, Lee et al., 1999). Within the case of ROCM debridements of included necrotic tissues frequently causes deforming, requiring evacuation of the sense of taste, nasal cartilage, and the orbit. These days endoscopic debridement is most considered due to the restricted tissue evacuation. In early aspiratory Mucormycosis patients were recuperated by lobectomy.

### 1.14.3. Combination Antifungal Therapy
In a patient with ROCM, a combination of amphotericin B and an echinocandin showed a successful outcome (Goldstein et al., 2009).

### 1.14.4. Hyperbaric Oxygen
Hyperbaric oxygen has been used in some patients with ROCM, but the benefit of this therapy has not been established. It represses the growth of fungus and also minimizes tissue hypoxia and acidosis which promotes vascular invasion by Mucorales (Ferguson et al., 1988).

## 2. Cryptococcosis

### 2.1. Introduction

Cryptococcosis is possibly an angio intrusive fungal infection caused by an encapsulated yeast Cryptococcus neoformans (Hussain et al., 2020). It is an opportunistic fungal pathogen that is strongly believed to spread to humans through proximity to pigeon droppings which act as a source for infectious propagule (Pal, M., and Bulto Giro Boru 2010). The fungal type is widely present in the environment and humans are exposed to such fungus while inhalation (Denham et al., 2018). Individuals with good immunocompetence troubleshoot the fungal infection and to an extent, they will have limited superficial infections which might be chronic. Immunocompromised people are most susceptible to cryptococcal infection (Maziarz et al., 2016). The disease is not contagious (Spread from one tainted individual to another). In most cases, the infection starts within the lungs (pulmonary form) and may then become disseminated via systemic circulation to the brain, skin, and bone and also affects the liver, kidney, heart, and even testis (Philip et al., 2012).

## 2.2. Causative Agent

The genus *Cryptococcus* encompasses nearly 50 species among them *C. neoformans* and *C. gatti* are considered major causes of infection (Ingavale et al., 2008; Buchanan and Murphy, 1998). Cryptococcus spp. is surrounded by a capsular polysaccharide, which is mainly composed of glucuronoxylomannan (GXM), the dominant capsular polysaccharide, and galactoxylomannan (GalXM).

The scientific classification of *C. neoformans*:

- *Kingdom:* Fungi
- *Phylum:* Basidiomycota
- *Class:* Tremellomycetes
- *Order:* Tremellales
- *Family:* Tremellaceae
- *Genus: Cryptococcus*
- *Species: Cryptococcus neoformans*

## 2.3. Sources of *C. neoformans*

*C. neoformans* are isolated from the avian habitat and it is prevalent in environmental and clinical settings (Marr et al., 2012). *C. neorformans* was isolated from a wide range of avian bird species including turkeys, chickens, parrots, budgerigars, munia birds, and canaries. Also, reported in animals like a macaw, swan, parakeet, Guenon monkey, fox, potoroo, and sheep. Thus domestic or wild animals and birds are the carriers for *C. neoformans* (Pal and Bulto Giro Boru2010).

*C. neoformans* is sub-classified into *C. neoformans* var. *grubii* (serotype A) and *C. neoformans* var. *neoformans* (serotype D) and are primarily related to AIDS patients. Serotypes A and D are isolated from natural sources like the debris of *Eucalyptus* spp., *T. catappa*, *Corymbias* spp., and *Ficus* spp. (Vélez and Escandón 2016; Escandón et al., 2010; Granados and Castañeda 2005; Byrnes et al., 2009).

## 2.4. Predisposing Factors

The individuals with diseases like immunosuppression due to AIDS, lymphomas (e.g., Hodgkin's lymphoma), sarcoidosis, liver cirrhosis, long term corticosteroid therapy, Solid Organ Transplantation (SOT), medications to treat rheumatoid arthritis, cancer chemotherapy, and Idiopathic CD4 lymphopenia are more susceptible to Cryptococcal infection (Lin et al., 2015).

## 2.5. Epidemiology of Cryptococcosis

### 2.5.1. Worldwide

The cryptococcal infection causes approximately 15% of AIDS-related mortality globally (Moeng et al., 2020). It is reported that nearly 2, 20, 000 cases are reported every year due to Cryptococcal meningitis, and among that the estimated death is 1, 81, 000 per year (Rajasingham et al., 2017). In the USA the opportunistic cryptococcal infection is said to be reduced to nearly 90% after the incidence of Anti Retroviral Therapy (ART) (Jarvis et al., 2009). At present the incidence of Cryptococcal meningitis is high in Sub-Saharan Africa, followed by Asia and the Pacific as the ART is not effectively escalated among the developing countries (Maziarz et al., 2016 Rajasingham et al., 2017).

### 2.5.2. India

The tropical climate of India prompts a reasonable environment for *C. neoformans,* and the onset of the AIDS pandemic (1981) is driven to incite increment within the number of cases detailed in Cryptococcosis amid the final decade (Beyrer and Chris 2021). In India, the prevalence of Cryptococcal infection is high in Karnataka than in other states of India. It is then followed by Tamil Nadu, Andhra Pradesh, West Bengal, Orissa, Bihar, and Pondicherry. Mostly it affected the middle-aged men of age group approximately 35. HIV predominant cases were dominant among the middle-aged groups.

### 2.5.3. Pathogenicity

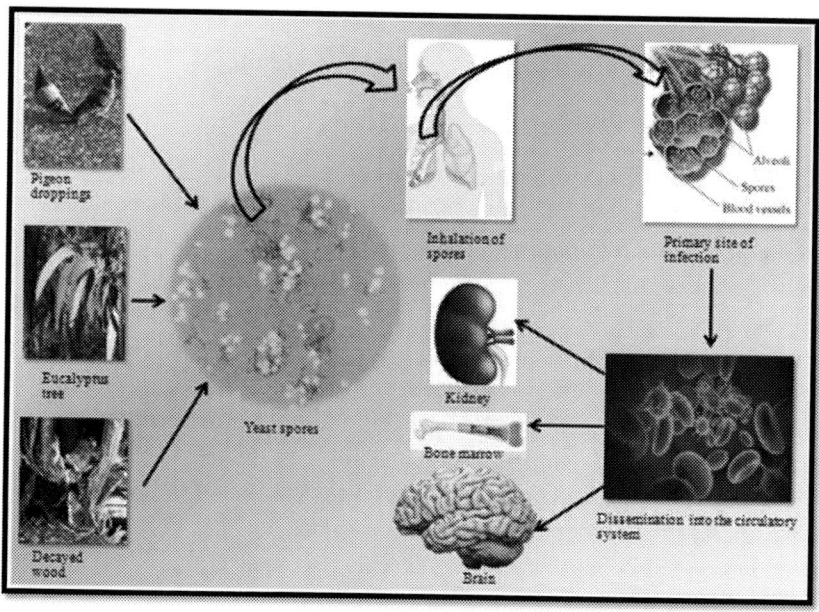

**Figure 3.** Pathogenesis of *C. neoformans*.

Inhalation of yeast spore causes it to deposit in pulmonary alveoli (survive in neutral to alkaline pH and physiological concentrations of carbon dioxide sometime recently phagocytosed by alveolar macrophages) (Pescador et al., 2020). Glucosylceramide synthase has been recognized as a striking factor in the survival of *C. neofomans* within the extracellular environment (Mitchell and Aaron 2006; Rittershaus et al., 2006). Unencapsulated yeast is readily phagocytosed and impeded considerably encapsulated yeast is more resistant to phagocytosis and other immune mechanisms. Encapsulated yeast causes modification of cellular organization, organelles result in accumulation of fungal material and interferes with phagolysosomal maturation, and cause disruption of the phagolysosomal membrane (Maziarz et al., 2016). Depolarization and fragmentation of mitochondria result in swelling and cytoskeleton abnormalities. Nonlytic exocytosis, vacuolation, and lytic exocytosis affect the inactivation of cell death pathways. As a sequel of metabolic modification, yeast extracellular vesicles cause disruption of intracellular architecture, accumulation of yeasts creating fungal masses Subversion of host immune response (Natural killer cells, Monocyte-derived macrophages, T lymphocytes) (Casadevall et al., 2018).

## 2.6. Genes Contributing to Virulence and Tolerance in *C. neoformans*

### 2.6.1. Virulence Genes in C. neoformans

There are approximately 184 virulence genes in *C. neoformans vargrubii, C. neoformans var neoformans*. Each protein serves to be responsible for increasing the virulence of *C. neoformans*. They all contribute to capsule synthesis, melanin production, and biofilm production. These genes help the organism tolerate heat, osmotic, and superoxide dismutase (SOD) stress. Phospholipase production by *Cryptococcus* may tend to disrupt human cell membranes. The enzymes like protease and urease are also considered to be toxic to the host. *ERG11* gene is responsible for the synthesis of 14α lanosterol demethylase, an important enzyme for sterol synthesis. *LAC1* and *LAC2* gene is responsible for the production of laccase enzyme that helps in melanin production and also inhibits phagocytic uptake (Orner et al., 2019). *CAP59*, *CAP10*, *CAP60*, *CAP64*, *CAS1*, *CXT1*, *KRE6*, *KTR3*, and *UGT1* are a few important genes that play a pivotal role in capsule synthesis and maintenance (Malachowski et al., 2016). Among various genes, *CHS3* gene is accountable for the synthesis of Chitin in the outer cell wall of fungi. *URE1*, *LAC1*, and *CAP59* are the three genes behind the production of biofilms. It is noted that Antiphagocytic protein 1 (*APP1*) and Laccase enzyme (*LAC1* and *LAC2*) are the predominant factors contributing to the virulence of *C. neoformans* (Orner et al., 2019).

### 2.6.2. Stress Tolerance Genes Contributing to Virulence

Among the various stress tolerance genes, autophagy-related genes are said to play a vital role in contributing to virulence. Autophagy is a catabolic process that helps the *Cryptococcus* to survive in nutrient-deficient conditions and various stress conditions.

**Table 3.** Autophagy related protein in *C. neoformans* (Zhao et al., 2019)

| S.no | Gene name | Function |
|---|---|---|
| 1. | ATG1 | Serine/ Threonine kinase (Matsuura et al., 1997) |
| 2. | ATG2 | Form a complex with ATG18; involved in ATG9 dynamics at PAS |
| 3. | ATG3 | Specific E2 enzyme for ATG8-PE formation |
| 4. | ATG4 | Cysteine protease and deconjugation enzyme; involved in the formation and cleavage of ATG8-PE |
| 5. | ATG5 | The target of ATG12 and interacts with ATG16 |
| 6. | ATG6 | Also known as Vsp30, a subunit of PI3K |
| 7. | ATG7 | Common E1 enzyme for ATG12- ATG5 and ATG8- PE formation |
| 8. | ATG8 | Ubiquitin-like protein conjugated to PE |
| 9. | ATG9 | Integral membrane protein |
| 10. | ATG11 | Acts as an adapter protein in selective autophagy |
| 11. | ATG12 | Ubiquitin-like protein and conjugated to ATG5 |
| 12. | ATG13 | Phosphorylated by TORC1 and regulates ATG1 activity |
| 13. | ATG14-03 | Recruits the PI3K complex to the PAS |
| 14. | ATG14-05 | Unknown |
| 15. | ATG15 | Encodes a putative lipase responsible for the disintegration of autophagic bodies |
| 16. | ATG16 | Required for the localization of ATG12-ATG5 to PAS |
| 17. | ATG18 | Binds to PI3P and regulates vacuole size |
| 18. | ATG20 | Sorting nexin family is required for organelle autophagy and contributes to general autophagy |
| 19. | ATG22 | Enables the reuse of the resulting macromolecules in the cytosol |
| 20. | ATG24 | Sorting nexin required for organelle autophagy; contributes to general autophagy |
| 21. | ATG26 | Essential for the degradation of very large methanol-induced Peroxisomes |
| 22. | ATG27 | The second transmembrane cycling protein; localizes to the Golgi |
| 23. | ATG101 | Unique subunit of the ATG1-ATG13 complex required in Mammals |

There are about 23 *ATG* genes in *C. neoformans*. Most of the *ATG*s positively regulates capsule production. Among them, *ATG1*, *ATG7*, *ATG8*, and *ATG9* promote good capsule growth. *ATG1*, *ATG7*, *ATG9*, *ATG11*, ATG16, and *ATG18* help in the survival of yeast during carbon starvation. ATG2, ATG9, *ATG16,* and *ATG 18* help in surviving nitrogen starvation conditions *ATG1, ATG2, ATG3, ATG4, ATG6, ATG8, ATG9, ATG13, ATG15, ATG16, ATG26,* and *ATG27* help in salt tolerance. *ATG2* and *ATG6* displayed higher sensitivity to oxidative stress caused by hydrogen peroxide, implying that these genes play essentially antioxidant roles. *ATG6, ATG7, ATG8, ATG12, ATG14-03, ATG20,* and *ATG 24* promote the growth of *C.*

*neoformans* at 37°C. *ATG6* and *ATG24* are considered to be essential for thermotolerance. *ATG2, ATG6, ATG14- 03,* and *ATG16* stimulate laccase production that promotes the production of melanin. ATG8 contribute to surviving starvation condition (Hu et al., 2008). *ATG11, ATG21, ATG31, ATG51, ATG61, ATG71, ATG91, ATG121, ATG14- 031, ATG14-051, ATG151* and *ATG18, ATG16, ATG 9,* and *ATG 2*contribute to the survival of the *Cryptococcus* spp. in the nitrogen depleted environment. *ATG111, ATG131, ATG14-031, ATG14-051, ATG151,* and *ATG201*helps to survive the glucose-depleted environment (Zhao et al., 2019).

## 2.7. Role of Genomics in *Cryptococcus* Diversification

The population structure analysis and genetic differentiation of *Cryptococcus* strains are based on their karyotypes, DNA fingerprints, Rapid amplified polymorphic DNA, Amplified fragment length polymorphism, and Intergenic spacer sequences of rDNA. The PCR-based techniques and DNA sequencing techniques expedited the strain classification. The MultiLocus Sequence Typing (MLST) is considered to be the standard technique for the classification of strains. It mainly uses the housekeeping genes of the organism for strain categorization. MLST has been proven to be a highly discriminatory technique for human pathogenic fungi classification. There are about six housekeeping genes in *Cryptococcus* spp. They are *CAP59* (capsular-associated protein), *GPD1* (glyceraldehyde- 3- phosphate dehydrogenase), *LAC1* (Laccase), *PLB1* (Phospholipase), *SOD1* (Cu, Zn superoxide dismutase), *URA5* (Orotidine monophosphate pyrophosphorylase) (Meyer et al., 2009). Among the six *CAP59* (polysaccharide capsules), *LAC1* (Melanin synthesis) and *PLB1* (cell invasion) were considered to promote virulence. The divergence in *URA 5* gene sequencing has classified *C. neoformans* into *C. neoformans var. grubii* and *C. neoformans var. neoformans*. The divergence among *C. neoformans* species have evolved approximately 50 million years ago (Franzot et al., 1999 Ngamskulrungroj et al.,2009).

Other than yeast form, *C. neoformans* exist in *MATa* and *MATα* mating sorts yeast cells within the environment (Lin, 2009). These mating types result in a filamentous cell type. Such dikaryon undergoes nuclear fusion, and meiosis and generates haploid spores. These haploid spores are inhaled by individuals from the environment and develop an infection in the respiratory system.

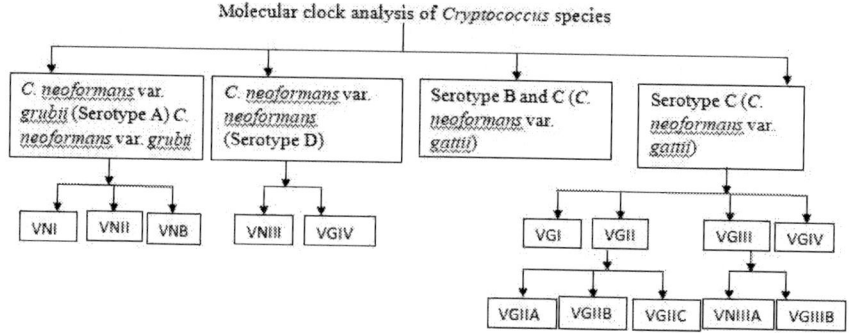

**Figure 4.** Molecular clock of *Cryptococcus* spp. (Kidd et al., 2004; Igreja et al., 2004; Byrnes et al., 2011; Byrnes et al., 2010).

## 2.8. Types of Cryptococcal Infection and Its Clinical Manifestations

*Cryptococcus neoformans* mainly affect the lungs as it enters the host via inhalation. Once it establishes infection in the lungs it will be disseminated via systemic circulation affecting other vital organs.

### 2.8.1. Cutaneous Cryptococcosis
Cutaneous cryptococcosis can be distinguished as either initial or secondary based on the mode of spread of the infection. It can be classified as localized or disseminated cryptococcosis (Noguchi et al., 2019). The symptoms include lesions (pustules, papules, nodular or ulcerated lesions), Skin rashes, petechiae (pinpoint red spots), bleeding in the skin, bruises and hardened plate- like patches (plaques).

### 2.8.2. Pulmonary Cryptococcosis
Pulmonary cryptococcosis is the primary opportunistic invasive infection that results in pneumonia-like illness (Setianingrum et al., 2019). The clinical manifestation includes non-productive cough, fatigue, chest pain, fever, segmental pneumonia resulting in fluid in the lungs and swollen lymph nodes (Setianingrum et al.,2019).

### 2.8.3. Cryptococcal Meningitis
It is a disseminated infection that spreads from the lungs to the brain. It is a result of cerebral edema and the symptoms include, Headache, fever, neck pain, nausea, vomiting, photophobia, diplopia, confusion or changes in behavior, depression, lethargy, agitation, cerebral edema might lead to

blindness, hydrocephalus, unusual sweating at night, ataxia, aphasia, seizures, and chorea (involuntary and unpredictable muscular movements) (Bicanic et al.,2004).

Inadvertent weight loss, appetite loss, stomach bloating, abdominal torment, abdominal swelling, weakness, bone pain or tenderness of breast bone, numbness/ tingling, and swollen glands are some of the symptoms when the cryptococcal infection becomes disseminated.

## 2.9. Complications

The complications of cryptococcosis are given in Figure 5.

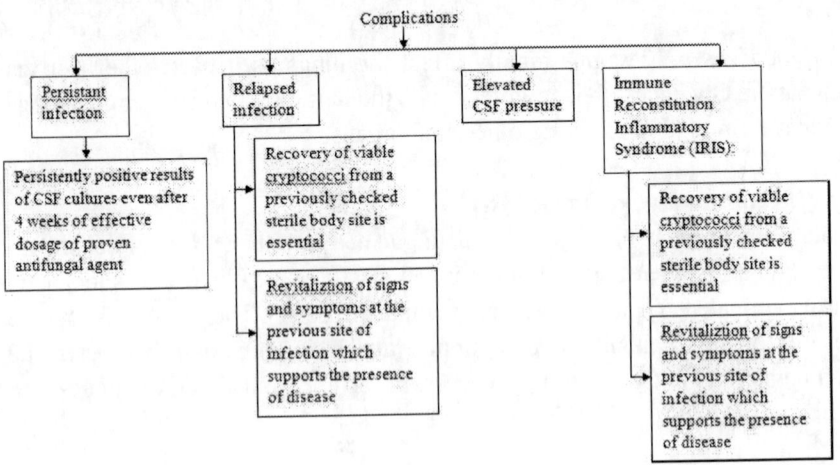

Figure 5. Complications of Cryptococcosis (Wiliamson et al., 2017).

## 2.10. Diagnosis Procedures

### 2.10.1 Physical Examination
Abnormal breath sounds, fast heart rate, fever, mental status changes, stiff neck, skin with papule, and ulcerative wound (Setianingrum et al., 2019).

### 2.10.2. Cultural Identification
In solid agar plates, the *Cryptococcus* culture appears as opaque, white to cream colonies. It takes nearly 48 to 72 hours to grow when the plates are

maintained at 30-35°C under aerobic conditions (Kwon-Chung et al., 1992). Birdseed agar is a selective and differential media for *Cryptococcus neoformans* where it grows as brown mucoid colonies. *Cryptococcus* produces an enzyme phenoloxidase a necessary enzyme for melanin production.

### 2.10.3. Microscopy
Indian ink staining (Preliminary test done directly from CFU sample for identification of capsule forming yeast), Grocott methenamine silver (GMS) staining, and fixed tissue specimen staining for capsule producing yeasts may too be recognized and affirmed as *C. neoformans* using positive mucicarmine or Masson-Fontana staining (Jarvis et al., 2008).

### 2.10.4. Antigen Detection
Antigen detection alludes to the rapid detection of antigen that has higher affectability than microscopy or culture. It incorporates the Latex Agglutination Test (LAT), Enzyme Immunoassay (EIA), and Lateral Flow Assay (LFA) (Chen et al., 2014, Mc Mullan et al., 2012).

### 2.10.5. Histopathology Analysis
*Cryptococcus* spp. is recognized by histologic staining of tissues from lungs, skin, brain, and other vital organs (Shibuya et al., 2002). Histopathologic staining of collected tissue is more delicate than the Indian ink staining strategy.

### 2.10.6. Diagnostic Imaging
Computed Tomography (CT), Magnetic Resonance Imaging (MRI), Bronchoscopy, Chest X-ray, and Positron Emission Tomography (Skiada et al., 2018).

## 2.11. Treatments

The treatment strategy for the *Cryptococcus* spp. infected patients vary based on their primary cause and the region of the body affected (Beardsley et al., 2019).

### 2.11.1. Patients with AIDS

All HIV-infected patients require treatment. For meningitis or severe aspiratory illness, the standard administration consists of the following:

#### 2.11.1.1. Induction Therapy for Severe Pulmonary or CNS Infection

Amphotericin B (0.7 to 1.0 mg/kg/day) + Flucytosine (100 mg/kg/day orally) or Amphotericin B + Fluconazole for 2 weeks. Liposomal amphotericin B (3 to 4 mg/kg/day) or Amphotericin B lipid complex (5 mg/kg/day) + flucytosine (100 mg/kg/day) for 2 weeks (Beardsley et al.,2019).

#### 2.11.1.2. Alternative Antifungal Combination during Induction Therapy

- Amphotericin B deoxycholate and fluconazole
- Fluconazole and flucytosine
- Fluconazole
- Itraconazole

### 2.11.2. Consolidation Therapy

Fluconazole (400 mg/day) is given for 7 to 8 weeks, but itraconazole at the same dose is satisfactory; however, itraconazole serum levels ought to be measured to form beyond any doubt that patients are retaining the drug (Beardsley et al., 2019).

### 2.11.3. Maintenance Therapy

Most HIV patients need maintenance therapy until CD4 cell counts are > 150/mcL. Fluconazole 200 mg/ day orally once a day is preferred for 1 or more years

#### 2.11.3.1. Alternative Antifungal Therapy during Maintenance Therapy

- Itraconazole (400 mg/day) is recommended for a prolonged period of 1 or more years
- Amphotericin B deoxycholate (1 mg/kg/week) for 1 or more years is suggested

### 2.11.4. Asymptomatic or Mild to Moderate Pulmonary Infections

Patients with mellow to direct side effects of the localized aspiratory association are treated with fluconazole 400 mg orally once a day for 6 to 12 months. The said antifungals have strong side impacts; consequently, the utilization must be observed.

### 2.11.5. Transplant Related Disease

#### 2.11.5.1. Induction Therapy
Liposomal amphotericin B is given at the dosage of 3 to 4 mg/kg/day or amphotericin B lipid complex is endorsed at the dosage of 5 mg/kg/day in combination with flucytosine at 100 mg/kg/day for 2 weeks.

#### 2.11.5.2. Induction Therapy Alternatives

- Either Liposomal amphotericin B (6 mg/kg/day) or amphotericin B lipid complex (5 mg/kg/day) are endorsed for a period of 4 to 6 weeks.
- Amphotericin B deoxycholate (0.7 mg/kg/day) for 4 to 6 weeks.

#### 2.11.5.3. Consolidation Therapy
Fluconazole is prescribed at the dosage of 400 to 800 mg/day for 8 weeks.

#### 2.11.5.4. Maintenance Therapy
Fluconazole is given at the dosage of 200 to 400 mg/day for 6 months to 1 year.

### 2.11.6. Patients without AIDS
Patients with pulmonary illness, skin with localized lesions, and lesions in bone are required to be treated with Fluconazole orally 200-400 mg once a day for 6 months to 12 months. In severe cases of the disease, amphotericin B 0.5 to 1.0 mg/Kg along with flucytosine 25 mg/Kg orally every 6 hours is given for several weeks.

### 2.11.7. Meningitis Patients

#### 2.11.7.1. Induction Therapy

- Induction therapy starts with the administration of amphotericin B deoxycholate 0.7 mg/kg IV once a day in combination with flucytosine 100 mg/kg/day orally

administered for 2 to 4weeks
- Liposomal amphotericin B (3 to 4 mg/kg/day) or amphotericin B lipid complex (5 mg/kg/day) in combination with flucytosine is preferred for 4 weeks. The combination of Amphotericin B and Flucytosine is considered to have the best antifungal action against Cryptococcus infection and it showed a greater survival rate over amphotericin alone. The major problem in using flucytosine is its cost. Due to its high cost, it is often unavailable in underdeveloped or developing regions where the disease burden issignificant.

*2.11.7.2. Consolidation Therapy*

Consolidation therapy is administered with fluconazole 400 mg orally once a day for 8 weeks.

*2.11.7.3. Maintenance Therapy*

The maintenance therapy with fluconazole 200 mg orally once a day for 6 to 12 months.

Repeated lumbar puncture is important to manage elevated opening pressures (Perfect et al., 2010; Perfect et al., 2015).

## 2.12. Cryptococcal Meningitis and COVID-19

It is an infrequent scenario where patients with COVID get co-infected with angio invasive *C. neoformans*. In such cases, cryptococcal infections are considered to be secondary fungal infections. It is mainly recorded in senior citizens above 60 years who got COVID infections with a previous history of complications such as Diabetes mellitus, Hypertension, Hydrocephalus, and encephalopathy. Cryptococcal meningitis is caused due to immune compression after treatment of COVID. *Cryptococcus* is an opportunistic pathogen it affects the patient post-COVID infection, increasing the complications leading to sepsis and mortality. Such cases were seen in extremely ill patients. The COVID recovered patients were tested positive for *Cryptococcus* via CSF antigen detection and Blood cultures. It is pivotal to avoid misdiagnosis and mismanagement, keeping in mind the high morbidity of COVID-19 patients, especially very ill ones or accompanied by the coinfections of fungi. It is salient to diagnose opportunistic infections like Cryptoccocal meningitis or Cryptococcaemia in the early stage in the immune-compromised patients who have a higher rate of mortality (Khatib et al.,2021).

## Conclusion

To summarize, Mucoromycosis and Cryptococcosis cause an alarming threat due to the increased state of immune compression among people around the world. Though the actual reason for the spread of these diseases is unknown it turns out to be the cause of the alarming mortality rate. The major condition to survive and manage catastrophic diseases is the early and exact diagnosis and usage of prompt therapeutic drugs at the prescribed dosage. The interdisciplinary studies on these angioinvasive fungal pathogens such as omics studies help to know the fungal genetic makeup, their expression of genes during the time of causing disease, mode of action of drugs on the target protein, etc. and will help to design new drugs with high efficiency and low toxicity so that the patient can survive the disease without the side effects of drugs.

## References

Abdollahi, Akram, TaherehShokohi, Nasrin Amirrajab, R. Poormosa, A. M. Kasiri, S. J. Motahari, S. M. Ghoreyshi et al. "Clinical features, diagnosis, and outcomes of rhino-orbito-cerebral Mucormycosis-A retrospective analysis." *Current Medical Mycology* 2, no. 4 (2016): 15.

Artis, William M., John A. Fountain, Harry K. Delcher, and Henry E. Jones. "A mechanism of susceptibility to Mucormycosis in diabetic ketoacidosis transferrin and iron availability." *Diabetes* 31, no. 12 (1982):1109-1114.

Beardsley, Justin, Tania C. Sorrell, and Sharon C-A. Chen. "Central nervous system cryptococcal infections in non-HIV infected patients." *Journal of Fungi* 5, no. 3 (2019): 71.

Beyrer, Chris. "A pandemic anniversary: 40 years of HIV/AIDS." *The Lancet* 397, no. 10290 (2021): 2142-2143.

Bicanic, Tihana, and Thomas S. Harrison. "Cryptococcal meningitis." *British Medical Bulletin* 72, no. 1 (2004): 99-118.

Binder, U., E. Maurer, and C. Lass-Flörl. "Mucormycosis–from the pathogens to the disease." *Clinical Microbiology and Infection* 20 (2014): 60-66.

Boelaert, Johan R., M. De Locht, J. Van Cutsem, V. Kerrels, B. Cantinieaux, A. Verdonck, H. W. Van Landuyt, and Yves-Jacques Schneider. "Mucormycosis during deferoxamine therapy is a siderophore-mediated infection. *In vitro* and *in vivo* animal studies." *The Journal of clinical investigation* 91, no. 5 (1993):1979-1986.

Buchanan KL, Murphy JW. What makes Cryptococcus neoformans a pathogen? *Emerg Infect Dis* 1998;4:71–83. doi:10.3201/eid0401.980109.

Byrnes EJ, Bartlett KH, Perfect JR, Heitman J. Cryptococcus gattii: an emerging fungal pathogen infecting humans and animals. *Microbes Infect* 2011;13:895–907.

Byrnes EJ, Bildfell RJ, Frank SA, Mitchell TG, Marr KA, Heitman J. Molecular Evidence That the Range of the Vancouver Island Outbreak of Cryptococcus gattii Infection Has Expanded into the Pacific Northwest in the United States. *J Infect Dis* 2009;199:1081–6.

Byrnes EJ, Li W, Lewit Y, Ma H, Voelz K, Ren P, et al. Emergence and Pathogenicity of Highly Virulent Cryptococcus gattii Genotypes in the Northwest United States. *PLoSPathog* 2010;6:e1000850.

Cánovas-Márquez, José Tomás, María Isabel Navarro-Mendoza, Carlos Pérez-Arques, Carlos Lax, GhizlaneTahiri, José Antonio Pérez-Ruiz, Damaris Lorenzo-Gutiérrez et al. "Role of the Non-Canonical RNAi Pathway in the Antifungal Resistance and Virulence of Mucorales." *Genes* 12, no. 4 (2021):586.

Chamilos, G., R. E. Lewis, G. Lamaris, T. J. Walsh, and D. P. Kontoyiannis. "Zygomycetes hyphae trigger an early, robust proinflammatory response in human polymorphonuclear neutrophils through toll-like receptor 2 induction but display relative resistance to oxidative damage." *Antimicrobial Agents and Chemotherapy* 52, no. 2 (2008): 722-724.

Chander, Jagdish, Mandeep Kaur, Nidhi Singla, R. P. S. Punia, Surinder K. Singhal, Ashok K. Attri, Ana Alastruey-Izquierdo, Alberto M. Stchigel, Jose F. Cano-Lira, and JosepGuarro. "Mucormycosis: battle with the deadly enemy over a five-year period in India." *Journal of Fungi* 4, no. 2 (2018): 46.

Chang, Miwha, Edward Sionov, Ami KhanalLamichhane, Kyung J. Kwon-Chung, and Yun C. Chang. "Roles of three Cryptococcus neoformans and Cryptococcus gattii efflux pump-coding genes in response to drug treatment." *Antimicrobial Agents and Chemotherapy* 62, no. 4 (2018): e01751-17.

Chen, Sharon C-A., Wieland Meyer, and Tania C. Sorrell. "Cryptococcus gattii infections." *Clinical Microbiology Reviews* 27, no. 4 (2014): 980-1024.

Chibucos, Marcus C., Sameh Soliman, TeclegiorgisGebremariam, Hongkyu Lee, Sean Daugherty, Joshua Orvis, Amol C. Shetty et al. "An integrated genomic and transcriptomic survey of Mucormycosis-causing fungi." *Nature Communications* 7, no. 1 (2016): 1-11.

Chinn, R. Y., and RICHARD D. Diamond. "Generation of chemotactic factors by Rhizopus oryzae in the presence and absence of serum: relationship to hyphal damage mediated by human neutrophils and effects of hyperglycemia and ketoacidosis." *Infection and Immunity* 38, no. 3 (1982):1123-1129.

Chowdhary, A., J. F. Meis, J. Guarro, Gs De Hoog, S. Kathuria, M. C. Arendrup, S. E., V.T., A.P. ArikanAkdagli et al. "ESCMID and ECMM joint clinical guidelines for the diagnosis and management of systemic phaeohyphomycosis: diseases caused by black fungi." *Clinical Microbiology and Infection* 20 (2014): 47-75.

Denham, Steven T., and Jessica Brown. "Mechanisms of pulmonary escape and dissemination by Cryptococcus neoformans." *Journal of Fungi* 4, no. 1 (2018): 25.

Eid, Rawan, Nagla TT Arab, and Michael T. Greenwood. "Iron mediated toxicity and programmed cell death: A review and a re-examination of existing paradigms." *Biochimica et Biophysica Acta (BBA)-Molecular Cell Research* 1864, no. 2 (2017): 399-430.

Escandón P, Sánchez A, Firacative C, Castañeda E. "Isolation of Cryptococcus gattii molecular type VGIII, from Corymbiaficifolia detritus in Colombia." *Med Mycol* 2010;48:675–8. doi:10.3109/13693780903420633.

Ferguson, Berrylin J., Thomas G. Mitchell, Richard Moon, Enrico M. Camporesi, and Joseph Farmer. "Adjunctive hyperbaric oxygen for treatment of rhinocerebral Mucormycosis." *Reviews of Infectious Diseases* 10, no. 3 (1988): 551-559.

Franzot SP, Salkin IF, Casadevall A. Cryptococcus neoformans var. grubii: Separate varietal status for Cryptococcus neoformans serotype A isolates. *J Clin Microbiol* 1999;37:838–40.

Gamaletsou, Maria N., Nikolaos V. Sipsas, Emmanuel Roilides, and Thomas J. Walsh. "Rhino-orbital-cerebral Mucormycosis." *Current Infectious Disease Reports* 14, no. 4 (2012):423-434.

Garcia, Alexis, Sandeep Vellanki, and Soo Chan Lee. "Genetic tools for investigating Mucorales fungal pathogenesis." *Current Clinical Microbiology Reports* 5, no. 3 (2018):173-180.

Goldstein, Ellie JC, Brad Spellberg, Thomas J. Walsh, Dimitrios P. Kontoyiannis, John Edwards Jr, and Ashraf S. Ibrahim. "Recent advances in the management of Mucormycosis: from bench to bedside." *Clinical Infectious Diseases* 48, no. 12 (2009): 1743-1751.

Granados DP, Castañeda E. "Isolation and characterization of Cryptococcus neoformans varieties recovered from natural sources in Bogotá, Colombia, and study of ecological conditions in the area." *MicrobEcol* 2005;49:282–90.

Gryganskyi, Andrii P., Jacob Golan, Somayeh Dolatabadi, Stephen Mondo, Sofia Robb, Alexander Idnurm, Anna Muszewska et al. "Phylogenetic and phylogenomic definition of Rhizopus species." *G3: Genes, Genomes, Genetics* 8, no. 6 (2018): 2007-2018.

Hernández, Jorge L., and Clifford J. Buckley. *Mucormycosis.* StatPearls Publishing: Florida. (2019).

Hoang, Kathy, Tony Abdo, J. Matthew Reinersman, Rufei Lu, and Nelson Iván AgudeloHiguita. "A case of invasive pulmonary Mucormycosis resulting from short courses of corticosteroids in a well-controlled diabetic patient." *Medical Mycology Case Reports* 29 (2020): 22-24.

Hoffmann, K., J. Pawłowska, G. Walther, M. Wrzosek, G. S. De Hoog, G. L. Benny, P. M. Kirk, and K. Voigt. "The family structure of the Mucorales: a synoptic revision based on comprehensive multigene-genealogies." *Persoonia-Molecular Phylogeny and Evolution of Fungi* 30, no. 1 (2013): 57-76.

Howard, Dexter H. "Acquisition, transport, and storage of iron by pathogenic fungi." *Clinical Microbiology Reviews* 12, no. 3 (1999): 394-404.

Hu, Guowu, Moshe Hacham, Scott R. Waterman, John Panepinto, Soowan Shin, Xiaoguang Liu, Jack Gibbons et al. "PI3K signaling of autophagy is required for starvation tolerance and virulenceof Cryptococcus neoformans." *The Journal of Clinical Investigation* 118, no. 3 (2008):1186-1197.

Hussain, K., Khalil, DharaMalavia, Elizabeth M Johnson, Jennifer Littlechild, C. Peter Winlove, Frank Vollmer, and Neil AR Gow. "Biosensors and diagnostics for fungal detection." *Journal of Fungi* 6, no. 4 (2020): 349.

Ibrahim, Ashraf S., Brad Spellberg, Thomas J. Walsh, and Dimitrios P. Kontoyiannis. "Pathogenesis of Mucormycosis." *Clinical Infectious Diseases* 54, no. suppl_1 (2012): S16-S22.

Ibrahim, Ashraf S., Teclegiorgis Gebremariam, Mingfu Liu, Georgios Chamilos, Dimitrios P. Kontoyiannis, Richard Mink, Kyung J. Kwon-Chung et al. "Bacterial endosymbiosis is widely present among zygomycetes but does not contribute to the pathogenesis of Mucormycosis." *The Journal of Infectious Diseases* 198, no. 7 (2008):1083-1090.

Igreja RP, Dos Santos Lazéra M, Wanke B, Gutierrez Galhardo MC, Kidd SE, Meyer W. "Molecular epidemiology of Cryptococcus neoformans isolates from AIDS patients of the Brazilian city, Rio de Janeiro." *Med Mycol* 2004;42:229-38.

Ingavale SS, Chang YC, Lee H, McClelland CM, Leong ML, Kwon-Chung KJ. Importance of mitochondria in survival of Cryptococcus neoformans under low oxygen conditions and tolerance to cobalt chloride. *PLoSPathog* 2008;4:e1000155. doi:10.1371/journal.ppat.1000155.

Jarvis, Joseph N., Andrew Boulle, Angela Loyse, Tihana Bicanic, Kevin Rebe, Anthony Williams, Thomas S. Harrison, and Graeme Meintjes. "High ongoing burden of cryptococcal disease in Africa despite antiretroviral roll out." *AIDS (London, England)* 23, no. 9 (2009): 1182.

Jarvis, Joseph N., and Thomas S. Harrison. "Pulmonary cryptococcosis." In *Seminars in Respiratory and Critical Care Medicine*, vol. 29, no. 02, pp. 141-150. © Thieme Medical Publishers, 2008.

Jeong, W., C. Keighley, R. Wolfe, W. Leng Lee, M. A. Slavin, D. C. M. Kong, and SC-A. Chen. "The epidemiology and clinical manifestations of *Mucor*mycosis: a systematic review and meta-analysis of case reports." *Clinical Microbiology and Infection* 25, no. 1 (2019): 26-34.

Jung, Won Hee, Anita Sham, Tianshun Lian, Arvinder Singh, Daniel J. Kosman, and James W. Kronstad. "Iron source preference and regulation of iron uptake in Cryptococcus neoformans." *PLoS Pathogens* 4, no. 2 (2008): e45.

Khatib, Mohamad Y., Amna A. Ahmed, Said B. Shaat, Ahmed S. Mohamed, and Abdulqadir J. Nashwan. "Cryptococcemia in a patient with COVID-19: A case report." *Clinical Case Reports* 9, no. 2 (2021): 853-855.

Kidd SE, Hagen F, Tscharke RL, Huynh M, Bartlett KH, Fyfe M, et al. A rare genotype of Cryptococcus gattii caused the cryptococcosis outbreak on Vancouver Island (British Columbia, Canada). *Proc Natl Acad Sci*2004;101:17258-63.

Kontoyiannis, Dimitrios P., Kieren A. Marr, Benjamin J. Park, Barbara D. Alexander, Elias J. Anaissie, Thomas J. Walsh, James Ito et al. "Prospective surveillance for invasive fungal infections in hematopoietic stem cell transplant recipients, 2001–

2006: overview of the Transplant-Associated Infection Surveillance Network (TRANSNET) Database." *Clinical Infectious Diseases* 50, no. 8 (2010): 1091-1100.

Kouadio, Isidore K., Syed Aljunid, Taro Kamigaki, Karen Hammad, and Hitoshi Oshitani. "Infectious diseases following natural disasters: prevention and control measures." *Expert Review of Anti-Infective Therapy* 10, no. 1 (2012):95-104.

Lackner, Nina, Wilfried Posch, and Cornelia Lass-Flörl. "Microbiological and molecular diagnosis of Mucormycosis: from old to new." *Microorganisms* 9, no. 7 (2021): 1518.

Lass-Flörl, C. "Zygomycosis: conventional laboratory diagnosis." *Clinical Microbiology and Infection* 15 (2009): 60-65.

Lax, Carlos, Carlos Pérez-Arques, María Isabel Navarro-Mendoza, José Tomás Cánovas-Márquez, GhizlaneTahiri, José Antonio Pérez-Ruiz, Macario Osorio-Concepción et al. "Genes, pathways, and mechanisms involved in the virulence of *Mucorales*." *Genes* 11, no. 3 (2020): 317.

Lin, Ying-Ying, Stephanie Shiau, and Chi-Tai Fang. "Risk factors for invasive Cryptococcus neoformans diseases: a case-control study." *PloS one* 10, no. 3 (2015): e0119090.

Malachowski, Antoni N., Mohamed Yosri, Goun Park, Yong-Sun Bahn, Yongqun He, and Michal A. Olszewski. "Systemic approach to virulence gene network analysis for gaining new insight into cryptococcal virulence." *Frontiers in Microbiology* 7 (2016):1652.

Matsuura, Akira, Miki Tsukada, Yoh Wada, and Yoshinori Ohsumi. "Apg1p, a novel protein kinase required for the autophagic process in Saccharomyces cerevisiae." *Gene* 192, no. 2 (1997): 245-250.

Maziarz, Eileen K., and John R. Perfect. "Cryptococcosis." *Infectious Disease Clinics* 30, no. 1 (2016): 179-206.

McMullan, Brendan J., Catriona Halliday, Tania C. Sorrell, David Judd, Sue Sleiman, Debbie Marriott, Tom Olma, and Sharon CA Chen. "Clinical utility of the cryptococcal antigen lateral flow assay in a diagnostic mycology laboratory." *PLoS One* 7, no. 11 (2012): e49541.

Meyer W, Aanensen DM, Boekhout T, Cogliati M, Diaz MR, Esposto MC, et al. Consensus multi-locus sequence typing scheme for Cryptococcus neoformans and Cryptococcus gattii. Med Mycol 2009.

Mitchell, Aaron P. "Cryptococcal virulence: beyond the usual suspects." *The Journal of Clinical Investigation* 116, no. 6 (2006): 1481-1483.

Moeng, Letumile R., James Milburn, Joseph N. Jarvis, and David S. Lawrence. "HIV-associated Cryptococcal Meningitis: a Review of Novel Short-Course and Oral Therapies." *Current Treatment Options in Infectious Diseases* 12, no. 4 (2020): 422-437.

Muqeetadnan, Mohammed, Ambreen Rahman, Syed Amer, Salman Nusrat, Syed Hassan, and Syed Hashmi. "Pulmonary *Mucormycosis*: an emerging infection." *Case Reports in Pulmonology* 2012 (2012).

Nagy, Gábor, Sándor Kiss, Rakesh Varghese, Kitti Bauer, Csilla Szebenyi, Sándor Kocsubé, Mónika Homa et al. "Characterization of three pleiotropic drug resistance transporter genes and their participation in the azole resistance of *Mucor circinelloides*." *Frontiers in Cellular and Infection Microbiology* 11 (2021):273.

Navarro-Mendoza, María Isabel, Carlos Pérez-Arques, Shweta Panchal, Francisco E. Nicolás, Stephen J. Mondo, Promit Ganguly, Jasmyn Pangilinan et al. "Early diverging fungus *Mucor circinelloides* lacks centromeric histone CENP-A and displays a mosaic of point and regional centromeres." *Current Biology* 29, no. 22 (2019): 3791-3802.

Neblett Fanfair, Robyn, Kaitlin Benedict, John Bos, Sarah D. Bennett, Yi-Chun Lo, Tolu Adebanjo, Kizee Etienne et al. "Necrotizing cutaneous Mucormycosis after a tornado in Joplin, Missouri, in 2011." *New England Journal of Medicine* 367, no. 23 (2012): 2214-2225.

Ngamskulrungroj P, Gilgado F, Faganello J, Litvintseva AP, Leal AL, Tsui KM, et al. Genetic Diversity of the Cryptococcus Species Complex Suggests that Cryptococcus gattii Deserves to Have Varieties. *PLoS One* 2009;4:e5862.

Noguchi, Hiromitsu, Tadahiko Matsumoto, Utako Kimura, MasataroHiruma, Masahiro Kusuhara, and Hironobu Ihn. "Cutaneous cryptococcosis." *Medical Mycology Journal* 60, no. 4 (2019):101-107.

Pal, M., and Bulto Giro Boru. "Natural habitat of Cryptococcus neoformans." *J Nat Hist* 6, no. 1 (2010): 5-8.

Pappas, Peter G., Barbara D. Alexander, David R. Andes, Susan Hadley, Carol A. Kauffman, Alison Freifeld, Elias J. Anaissie et al. "Invasive fungal infections among organ transplant recipients: results of the Transplant-Associated Infection Surveillance Network (TRANSNET)." *Clinical Infectious Diseases* 50, no. 8 (2010): 1101-1111.

Park, Benjamin J., Peter G. Pappas, Kathleen A. Wannemuehler, Barbara D. Alexander, Elias J. Anaissie, David R. Andes, John W. Baddley et al. "Invasive non-Aspergillus mold infections in transplant recipients, United States, 2001–2006." *Emerging Infectious Diseases* 17, no. 10 (2011): 1855.

Pérez, A. D. C., & Welsh, E. C. (2017). Ivett Miranda, et al. "Cutaneous Mucormycosis.". *An Bras Dermatol*, 92(3), 304-311.

Pérez-Arques, Carlos, María Isabel Navarro-Mendoza, Laura Murcia, Eusebio Navarro, VictorianoGarre, and Francisco Esteban Nicolás. "A non-canonical RNAi pathway controls virulence and genome stability in Mucorales." *PLoS Genetics* 16, no. 7 (2020): e1008611.

Perfect, John R., and Tihana Bicanic. "Cryptococcosis diagnosis and treatment: What do we know now." *Fungal Genetics and Biology* 78 (2015): 49-54.

Perfect, John R., William E. Dismukes, Francoise Dromer, David L. Goldman, John R. Graybill, Richard J. Hamill, Thomas S. Harrison et al. "Clinical practice guidelines for the management of cryptococcal disease: 2010 update by the Infectious Diseases Society of America." *Clinical Infectious Diseases* 50, no. 3 (2010): 291-322.

Pescador Ruschel, M. A., and B. Thapa. *Cryptococcal Meningitis*. StatPearls Publishing: Florida (2020).

Philip, Kandathil Joseph, Rupinder Kaur, Mohan Sangeetha, Kanwal Masih, Navjot Singh, and Anna Mani. "Disseminated cryptococcosis presenting with generalized lymphadenopathy." *Journal of Cytology/Indian Academy of Cytologists* 29, no. 3 (2012):200.

Prakash, Hariprasath, and Arunaloke Chakrabarti. "Epidemiology of Mucormycosis in India." *Microorganisms* 9, no. 3 (2021): 523.

Prakash, Hariprasath, Shivaprakash MandyaRudramurthy, Prasad S. Gandham, Anup Kumar Ghosh, Milner M. Kumar, Chandan Badapanda, and Arunaloke Chakrabarti. "Apophysomyces variabilis: draft genome sequence and comparison of predictive virulence determinants with other medically important Mucorales." *BMC Genomics* 18, no. 1 (2017): 1-13.

Priya, Poorna, Vithiya Ganesan, T. Rajendran, and V. G. Geni. "*Mucor*mycosis in a tertiary care center in South India: a 4-year experience." *Indian Journal Of Critical Care Medicine: Peer-Reviewed, Official Publication of Indian Society of Critical Care Medicine* 24, no. 3 (2020): 168.

Rajasingham, Radha, Rachel M. Smith, Benjamin J. Park, Joseph N. Jarvis, Nelesh P. Govender, Tom M. Chiller, David W. Denning, Angela Loyse, and David R. Boulware. "Global burden of disease of HIV-associated cryptococcal meningitis: an updated analysis." *The Lancet Infectious Diseases* 17, no. 8 (2017): 873-881.

Ribes, Julie A., Carolyn L. Vanover-Sams, and Doris J. Baker. "Zygomycetes in human disease." *Clinical Microbiology Reviews* 13, no. 2 (2000): 236-301.

Rittershaus, Philipp C., Talar B. Kechichian, Jeremy C. Allegood, Alfred H. Merrill, Mirko Hennig, Chiara Luberto, and Maurizio Del Poeta. "Glucosylceramide synthase is an essential regulator of pathogenicity of Cryptococcus neoformans." *The Journal of Clinical Investigation* 116, no. 6 (2006):1651-1659.

Roden, Maureen M., Theoklis E. Zaoutis, Wendy L. Buchanan, Tena A. Knudsen, Tatyana A. Sarkisova, Robert L. Schaufele, Michael Sein et al. "Epidemiology and outcome of zygomycosis: a review of 929 reported cases." *Clinical Infectious Diseases* 41, no. 5 (2005):634-653.

Sarrami, Amir Hossein, Mehrdad Setareh, Masoud Izadinejad, Noushin Afshar-Moghaddam, Mohammad Mehdi Baradaran-Mahdavi, and Mohsen Meidani. "Fatal disseminated Mucormycosis in an immunocompetent patient: a case report and literature review." *International Journal of Preventive Medicine* 4, no. 12 (2013): 1468.

Schrödl, Wieland, TiloHeydel, Volker U. Schwartze, Kerstin Hoffmann, AnkeGroße-Herrenthey, Grit Walther, Ana Alastruey-Izquierdo et al. "Direct analysis and identification of pathogenic Lichtheimia species by matrix-assisted laser desorption ionization–time of flight analyzer-mediated mass spectrometry." *Journal of Clinical Microbiology* 50, no. 2 (2012): 419-427.

Setianingrum, Findra, Riina Rautemaa-Richardson, and David W. Denning. "Pulmonary cryptococcosis: a review of pathobiology and clinical aspects." *Medical Mycology* 57, no. 2 (2019):133-150.

Singh, Awadhesh Kumar, Ritu Singh, Shashank R. Joshi, and Anoop Misra. "Mucormycosis in COVID-19: a systematic review of cases reported worldwide and in India." *Diabetes & Metabolic Syndrome: Clinical Research & Reviews* 15, no. 4 (2021): 102146.

Sipsas, Nikolaos V., Maria N. Gamaletsou, Amalia Anastasopoulou, and Dimitrios P. Kontoyiannis. "Therapy of Mucormycosis." *Journal of Fungi* 4, no. 3 (2018): 90.

Skiada, A., L. I. V. I. O. Pagano, A. Groll, S. Zimmerli, B. Dupont, KatrienLagrou, C. Lass-Florl et al. "Zygomycosis in Europe: analysis of 230 cases accrued by the registry of the European Confederation of Medical Mycology (ECMM) Working Group on Zygomycosis between 2005 and 2007." *Clinical Microbiology and Infection* 17, no. 12 (2011): 1859-1867.

Skiada, Anna, IoannisPavleas, and Maria Drogari-Apiranthitou. "Epidemiology and diagnosis of Mucormycosis: an update." *Journal of Fungi* 6, no. 4 (2020): 265.

Spellberg, Brad. "Gastrointestinal Mucormycosis: an evolving disease." *Gastroenterology & Hepatology* 8, no. 2 (2012): 140.

Spellberg, Brad, John Edwards Jr, and Ashraf Ibrahim. "Novel perspectives on Mucormycosis: pathophysiology, presentation, and management." *Clinical Microbiology Reviews* 18, no. 3 (2005): 556-569.

Stanford, Felicia Adelina, and Kerstin Voigt. "Iron assimilation during emerging infections caused by opportunistic fungi with emphasis on Mucorales and the development of antifungal resistance." *Genes* 11, no. 11 (2020): 1296.

Suganya, Ramalingam, Narasimhan Malathi, Vinithra Karthikeyan, and Vyshnavi Devi Janagaraj. "*Mucor*mycosis: a brief review." *J Pure Appl Microbiol* 13, no. 1 (2019): 161-165.

Thieken, Andrea, and Günther Winkelmann. "Rhizoferrin: a complexone type siderophore of the mocorales and entomophthorales (Zygomycetes)." *FEMS Microbiology Letters* 94, no. 1-2 (1992):37-41.

Tissot, Frederic, Samir Agrawal, Livio Pagano, Georgios Petrikkos, Andreas H. Groll, Anna Skiada, Cornelia Lass-Flörl, Thierry Calandra, Claudio Viscoli, and Raoul Herbrecht. "ECIL-6 guidelines for the treatment of invasive candidiasis, aspergillosis and Mucormycosis in leukemia and hematopoietic stem cell transplant patients." *Haematologica* 102, no. 3 (2017): 433.

Vélez N, Escandón P. "Distribution and association between environmental and clinical isolates of cryptococcus neoformans in Bogotá-Colombia, 2012-2015." *Mem Inst Oswaldo Cruz* 2016;111:642–8.

Waldorf, A. R. "Pulmonary defense mechanisms against opportunistic fungal pathogens." *Immunology Series* 47 (1989): 243-271.

Waldorf, A. R., N. Ruderman, and R. D. Diamond. "Specific susceptibility to Mucormycosis in murine diabetes and bronchoalveolar macrophage defense against Rhizopus." *The Journal of Clinical Investigation* 74, no. 1 (1984): 150-160.

Williamson PR, Jarvis JN, Panackal AA, Fisher MC, Molloy SF, Loyse A, Harrison TS. "Cryptococcal meningitis: epidemiology, immunology, diagnosis and therapy." *Nat Rev Neurol*. 2017Jan;13(1):13-24.

Xu, Qing, Yongqian Fu, Shuang Li, Ling Jiang, Guan Rongfeng, and He Huang. "Integrated transcriptomic and metabolomic analysis of Rhizopus oryzae with different morphologies." *Process Biochemistry* 64 (2018): 74-82.

Zaman, Kamran, Shivaprakash MandyaRudramurthy, Ashim Das, Naresh Panda, Prasanna Honnavar, Harsimran Kaur, and Arunaloke Chakrabarti. "Molecular diagnosis of rhino-orbito-cerebral Mucormycosis from fresh tissue samples." *Journal of Medical Microbiology* 66, no. 8 (2017):1124-1129.

Zhao, Xueru, Weijia Feng, Xiangyang Zhu, Chenxi Li, Xiaoyu Ma, Xin Li, Xudong Zhu, and Dongsheng Wei. "Conserved autophagy pathway contributes to stress tolerance and virulence and differentially controls autophagic flux upon nutrient starvation in Cryptococcus neoformans." *Frontiers in Microbiology* (2019):2690.

Zhao, Xueru, Weijia Feng, Xiangyang Zhu, Chenxi Li, Xiaoyu Ma, Xin Li, Xudong Zhu, and Dongsheng Wei. "Conserved autophagy pathway contributes to stress tolerance and virulence and differentially controls autophagic flux upon nutrient starvation in Cryptococcus neoformans." *Frontiers in Microbiology* (2019):2690.

Chapter 2

# Interdisciplinary Mathematical Modeling Approaches for Infectious Diseases

Gottumukkala Sai Bhavani[1],
Sumathi Kalankariyan[1],
Lavanya Sargunam[2]
and Anbumathi Palanisamy[1,*]

[1]Department of Biotechnology,
National Institute of Technology Warangal,
Telangana State, India
[2]Department of Mathematics,
Anna University, Chennai, Tamilnadu, India

## Abstract

An introductory overview on the mathematical modeling approaches for infectious diseases is discussed. Different types of models in epidemic spreading of the diseases along with their predicted mitigation strategies and their effectiveness are presented with relevant examples. The insightful predictions from mathematical modeling and analysis often contribute for understanding the dynamics, pattern of disease spread, predict, or develop effective treatment and quarantine or control strategies.

**Keywords**: mathematical modeling, Infectious disease, SIR models, epidemic spreading, pathogen spreading

---

[*] Corresponding Author's Email: anbu@nitw.ac.in.

In: Interdisciplinary Approaches on Opportunistic Infections ...
Editors: Jayapradha Ramakrishnan and Ganesh Babu Malli Mohan
ISBN: 978-1-68507-984-0
© 2022 Nova Science Publishers, Inc.

## Abbreviations

SIR – Susceptible Infectious Removal
IBM – Individual Based Model
IAV – Influenza A virus
PCF – Periciliary Fluid
HRT – Human Respiratory Tract
PDE – Partial Differential Equation
EVD – Ebola virus disease
SEIR – Susceptible Exposed Infected Recovered
NSFD – Non-Standard Finite Difference
ETR - Effective Transmission Rate

## 1. Introduction

History of the humankind has been influenced by many infectious diseases. Factors associated with disease spread such as spatial patterns, disease spread rates, subpopulations have displayed significant impact on the society. Disease patterns have been classified into endemic, outbreak, epidemic and pandemic by World Health Organization (WHO) (Prevention, 2018). Endemic is a disease that confines to a population; epidemic is uncontrolled rise in infection in a selected geographic location and pandemic is an endemic with no geographical limitations. Tracking of such epidemics, pandemics spread, their dynamics and patterns will contribute towards better public interventions. Mathematical models of infectious disease can assist in the process of tracking the disease dynamics and pattern of an epidemic / pandemic spread for public health interventions. Numerous such models have proven to be extremely valuable. The importance and practical applications of various types of mathematical models and predictions were evidently observed during the present COVID pandemic starting from December 2019. Mathematical models have become inevitable versatile tools to predict the rise and fall of the multiple waves of the pandemic, effect of vaccination, possibility of herd immunity and regulated/ controlled global travel.

Historically mathematical modeling and analysis of infectious disease spread has played key roles (i) in determining several strategies for disease spread; (ii) to generate and verify hypothesis and (iii) to determine the effect of various mitigation strategies. One of the first mathematical models for smallpox was developed by Daniel Bernoulli in 1760 to track the effectiveness of variolation (equivalent to modern day vaccination) in a healthy population (Hethcote, 2000). The classical triad model (Figure 1) for epidemiological spread consists of an external agent that causes the disease, a susceptible host and an environment that brings the possible interaction between host and agent. Bacteria, viruses, fungi, protozoa, and parasites are known causative biological agents for these infectious diseases and is transmitted through many modes (direct and indirect). From time immemorial infectious diseases has remained a cause for high morbidity and mortality. Numerous such incidences from prehistoric time until the present time have been identified and accounted (Piret & Boivin, 2021). Some examples with evidence include Plague of Athens (430 BC), Plague of Justinian (541-543 BCE), the Black Death (1346-1353) caused by *Yersinia pestis*, Multiple occurrences of Cholera pandemic of 18$^{th}$century, Spanish Flu (1918-1920),Polio epidemic of 19th -early 20th century, Asian Flu (1957-1959), Philadelphia yellow fever (1973), influenza A (H1N1) virus pandemic (2009-2010), West African Ebola Epidemic (2014-2016), Zika-virus Pandemic of South& central America by *Aedes* mosquitos (2015-Present) and recent SARS-Co-V2 outbreak (2019-Present)which is most recent (Piret & Boivin, 2021). Mathematical and Computational Epidemiology models have severed as a versatile tool to deal with many such epidemics and pandemics.

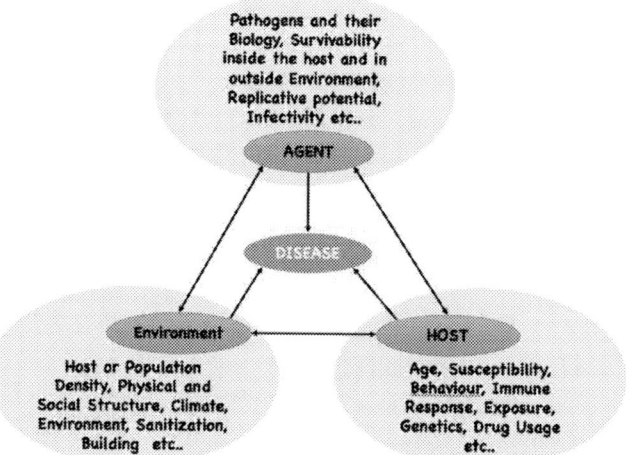

**Figure 1.** Classical trial model of epidemiological disease spread.
This consists of an agent, host and environment which might all influence the manner in which the disease spread may occur.

During epidemics, infectious disease pathogens are commonly transmitted between same species (human to human) or across species (e.g., animal to human). Transmission of a pathogen can occur directly between the hosts or indirectly through the intermediate hosts or the environment (Grassly & Fraser, 2008). Infectiousness and susceptibility are the key determinants of the efficiency of disease transmission (Grassly & Fraser, 2008). Infectiousness is a property of the host which encompass the host's ability to carry and transmit the pathogens to other individuals. Duration of infectiousness is a critical parameter to determine effective control measures (Cevik et al., 2021). Susceptibility is related to the exposure of the pathogens (from a host or intermediate) to the individuals who are not infected before. Depending on various factors such as the individual's immune response, previous exposure to the pathogen in the form of a vaccine, age, environment etc. will be key determinant of susceptibility. Depending on these factors the Susceptible individuals might become (i) infectious and spread the disease; (ii) can resist infection (if the vaccinated or if their immune system is strong) and (iii) spread the infectious disease without any visible or detectable symptoms.

Understanding the biology, behavior of pathogen and its transmission within the host and in environment is crucial for modeling and analysis of disease spread (Grassly & Fraser, 2008). The characteristics of the pathogens like (i) its replication potential and spreading withing the infected host; (ii) virulence; (iii) sensitivity to drug (if available) and (iv) its interaction with the genetic determinants of the host are key determinant of not only for the spread of the disease but also for identifying the parameters of the models (Grassly & Fraser, 2008). The following characteristic of the pathogen lays the route for its transmission. There are six main ways of transmission which are (i) Direct contact transmission through bodily fluids; (ii) Fomite transmission through inanimate objects; (iii) Airborne/Aerosol transmission through small droplets; (iv) Oral transmission though contaminated food or water; (v) vector borne transmission e.g., Malaria thorough mosquitos and (vi) Zoonotic transmission by switching from animals to human hosts e.g., COVID-19. For a Transmission to occur the following three components are essential: An Infected Individual, Susceptible Individual, and the effective contact between them depends on one of the above routes of transmissions. The transmission of the disease from infected individual to susceptible individual is referred to as transmission cycle. Many of the pathogens have a common life cycle that follows 3 phases within the host including Growth, Reproduction and Transmission (Despommier & Karapelou, 2012). For example, the process of parasite transmission and its assessment using various compartment models were reviewed elsewhere (White et al., 2018). Thus, understanding the biology and routes of transmission of pathogens are crucial for any disease spread.

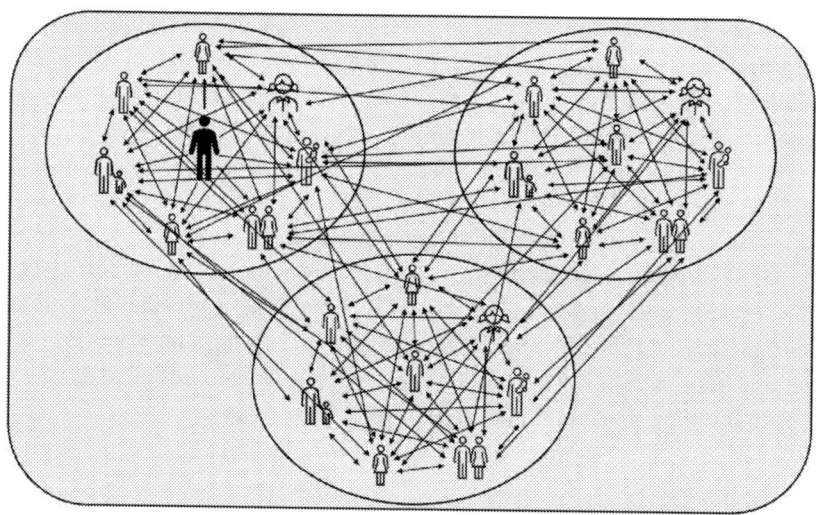

**Figure 2.** Network representation of disease spread within and across communities. Here we observe three representative community, individuals are nodes of the network. The arrows or edges represent the contact and possible transmission of disease through various routes. The shaded individual within one of the communities is a presentation of a super-spreader with or without symptoms.

Understanding the routes of transmission helps to explore, find, or develop and predict effective treatment or preventive strategies during the spread of the disease. Disrupting transmission is key to control and prevent infection. Disease transmission is a stochastic process (Grassly & Fraser, 2008). Data for disease transmission is usually obtained from government records, health and public databases. Patterns deciphered from the collected data determine the transmission rate for various air borne pathogens like influenza (Mikolajczyk & Kretzschmar, 2008). Hence it is important for scientific communities to have access to data on past and present disease spread. All models developed are simplifications of reality (Huppert & Katriel, 2013). Pathogens evolve, similarly mathematical models have evolved with rise in technological advancements in the fields computations and mathematical analysis leading to uncover the influence of pathogens on the larger ecology and vice versa. Integration of mathematical with statistical methods allows for estimation of the key parameters based on available data

(Grassly & Fraser, 2008). In the absence of data, models can be utilized to develop data collection strategies based on the hypothesis predicted by the models (Grassly & Fraser, 2008). Disease surveillance data based Mathematical modeling utilized for developing scientific hypothesis as well as disease control policy (Grassly & Fraser, 2008; Willem et al., 2017). Models analyze various such interventions and their possible outcomes to suggest strategic plan for implementation.

Apart from pathogen and its characteristics such as infection rate, viral load, life cycle etc. Environment such as the community structure, change in temperature, Individual behavior and group behavior within the environment is crucial. An individual within the community may contribute for super spreading (Figure 2) depending on their role and contact with other individuals or community and thus increasing the Effective Transmission Rate (ETR) of the disease spread. Indicative of such a super spreader is represented as shaded individual within the community in Figure 2.

## 2. SIR Models for Disease Spread

Infectious diseases are often analyzed using simple compartmental models. The population is assigned compartments and individuals progress between compartments are tracked and analyzed to understand the spread and recovery rates. These models predict information on how disease spreads, total number of infected/recovered, duration of epidemic and various epidemiological features. One such model is Susceptible-Infected-Recovered model (SIR) model which is a basic compartmental model. It consists of three compartments namely Susceptible (S), Infected (I), and Recovered (R) representing the health states. **S** represents the individuals that contracts the disease from infectious individuals and transfers to infectious compartments, while I represent infected compartment and R the total number of recovered or resistant population. The variables S, I, R represent the total number of individuals in the compartments. The first SIR model was developed by Kermack and McKendrick (1927) by assuming fixed population (Kermack & McKendrick, 1927).

$$\frac{dS}{dt} = \frac{-\beta * I * S}{N} \qquad (1)$$

$$\frac{dI}{dt} = \frac{\beta * I * S}{N} - \gamma * I \qquad (2)$$

$$\frac{dR}{dt} = \gamma * I \quad (3)$$

$$\frac{dS}{dt} + \frac{dI}{dt} + \frac{dR}{dt} = 0 \quad (4)$$

$$S(t) + T(t) + R(t) = N \quad (5)$$

where N is the total or entire population, β is the average number of contacts per person per time, if an individual is infectious for an average time period D, then γ = 1/D.

The disease spread dynamics depends on the ratio called as basic reproduction number given as $R_0$ and it can be taken as the ratio of $\frac{\beta}{\gamma}$. $R_o$ is crucial in determining the expected number of secondary infections and results from the single infected individual in the susceptible population (refer Equation 1 to understand the influence of contact on $R_o$). An epidemic can only occur if the reproduction number R is greater than 1. This threshold property provides information on potential for disease transmission and impact of disease control (Grassly & Fraser, 2008). Various methods used to estimate $R_o$, its practical use during the 2009 influenza-A (H1N1) virus pandemic and its importance is elaborately analyzed (Ridenour et al., 2014). It helps to understand the public outbreak and prepared public health response (Ridenour et al., 2014) which was evident during the current COVID-19 pandemic. Force of infection can be given by F = β * I, but for large populations it could be taken as F = β * I /Ns. In a model where every individual gets infected SIR model reduces to a simple SI model when there is no removal from the infectious compartment (γ=0) and follows a logistic solution.

One of the main assumptions of classic SIR models it that there is homogeneous mixing of I and S population, and the total population is constant over time (given by eqn (4)) which contradicts reality of varying population size. Also, SIR models consider infectivity β and recovery γ to be constant while in reality both depends on the period of infection which was observed to be a poison distribution with exponentially distributed means (Grassly & Fraser, 2008). Hence stochastic SIR models were explored to capture the random events and influences. There are numerous variations introduced to the basic SIR models to account for various factors influencing the spread of the infections. Many of these have made specific contribution in understating the emergence of disease and effectiveness of the controlling strategies.

## 3. Modified SIR Models for Disease Spread

There are numerous variations to classic SIR based modeling strategy which accounts for certain crucial factors that impacts disease spread. Modified SIR models attempt to quantify disease spread by accounting for specific characteristic signature of the disease spread which has provided different perspective and additional insights. Table 1 below provides detailed account of such modifications and their role in understanding the disease spread.

**Table 1.** Modified SIR models and their role in accounting for additional disease spread mechanisms

| Model | Variables | Specifics | References |
|---|---|---|---|
| SIR without vital Dynamics | | A classic SIR model which does not consider the dynamics of Birth and death, Demography related information is often omitted | (Capistrán et al., 2012; Giubilei, 2020; Harko & Mak, 2020; Hethcote, 1978; Kutrolli et al., 2020; Kuznetsov & Piccardi, 1994; Letsa-Agbozo et al., 2016; Monteiro & Mazorche, 2021) |
| SIR with vital Dynamic and population | | A Classic SIR model that accounts for Birth rate and mortality rate | (Adda & Bichara, 2011; Chen, 2020; Hethcote, 2009; Hill & Longini, 2003; Letsa-Agbozo et al., 2016; Li et al., 2015; Monteiro & Mazorche; Muñoz-Fernández et al., 2021) |
| SIS | Susceptible -> Infectious -> susceptible | Models that considered recovered individuals are susceptible for reinfection due to lack of immunity after recovery | (Allen, 1994; Balzotti et al., 2020; Bichara et al., 2014; Bichara et al., 2015; Castillo-Chavez et al., 2002; Hethcote & van den Driessche, 1995; Hethcote & Van Den Driessche, 2000; Li et al., 2007; Li & Cui, 2009; Meng et al., 2016; Menon et al., 2020; Ribassin-Majed & Lounes, 2010; Sanz et al., 2014; Zhang & Liu, 2009) |

| Model | Variables | Specifics | References |
|---|---|---|---|
| SIRD | Susceptible -> Infectious -> Recovered -> Deceased | Models that differentiate between Recovered and Diseased induvial | (Al-Raeei, 2020; Mohammadi et al., 2021; Tulu et al., 2017; Wang & Jia, 2019; Zewdie & Gakkhar, 2020) |
| SIRV | Susceptible -> Infectious -> Recovered -> Vaccinated | Models that take into consideration the vaccination of susceptible populations | (Ameen et al., 2020; Arachchi & Hasanthika; Cai et al., 2017; Ishikawa, 2018; Ma & Yu, 2020; Rifhat et al., 2021; Vardavas et al., 2007; Zhao & Yuan, 2016; Zhao et al., 2016) |
| MSIR | Maternally derived immunity -> Susceptible -> Infectious -> Recovered | Models that account for the passive immunity (Maternally derived Immunity) | (Bichara et al., 2014; Blaizot et al., 2019; Cador et al., 2016; Fajar & Liver, 2019; Menon et al., 2020) |
| SEIR | Susceptible -> Exposed -> Infectious -> Recovered | Models that considera latency period (Exposed) where individuals are exposed to the infection priorly across subpopulations | (Amira; Torres, 2018; Andrade & Duggan, 2020; Berger et al., 2020; Biswas et al., 2014; Bjørnstad et al., 2020; Cador et al., 2016; Dukic et al., 2012; Getz et al., 2019; Kuznetsov & Piccardi, 1994; Lekone & Finkenstädt, 2006; Olaniyi et al., 2020; Pandey et al., 2020; Syafruddin & Noorani, 2012; Umar et al., 2021; Yang et al., 2020) |
| SEIS | Susceptible -> Exposed -> Infectious -> susceptible | Similar to SEIR model however no immunity is achieved in the end | (Fan et al., 2001; Guo et al., 2010; Liu, 2017; Meng et al., 2013; Menon et al., 2020; Naim et al., 2021; Wan & Cui, 2007; Xu, 2012; Yang, 2016) |
| SEIRS | Susceptible -> Exposed -> Infectious -> Recovered -> susceptible | Considers the practical constraint that theRecovered individuals from SEIR module are susceptible to infection again due to lack of immunity | (Apenteng & Ismail, 2014; Bjørnstad et al., 2020; Cooke & van den Driessche, 1996; Denphedtnong et al., 2013; Gao et al., 2007; Greenhalgh, 1997; Jia & Xiao, 2018; Jiang et al., 2016; Jiao et al., 2008; Liu & Zhang, 2011; Liu et al., 1987; Mateus et al., 2017; Meng et al., 2007; Song et al., 2019; Trawicki, 2017; |

**Table 1.** (Continued)

| Model | Variables | Specifics | References |
|---|---|---|---|
| | | | Yu et al., 2021; Zhang & Si, 2014) |
| MSEIR | Maternally derived immunity -> Susceptible -> Exposed -> Infectious -> Recovered | SIR model with passive immunity and latency period | (Almeida et al., 2019; Anguelov et al., 2009; Bjørnstad et al., 2020; Gbolahan, 2010; Inaba, 2006; Menon et al., 2020; Momoh et al., 2011; Qureshi & Yusuf, 2019; Totaro, 2008) |
| MSEIRS | Maternally derived immunity -> Susceptible -> Exposed -> Infectious -> Recovered -> Susceptible | MSEIR model with low immunity or immunity lost after the R Stage | (Menon et al., 2020) |
| Carrier State | | Individuals sometimes recover but do not recover completely from the infection and move in and out of infectious compartment. Thus, are prone to act as carries for further infection | (Arif et al., 2019; Bronsvoort et al., 2016; Cao et al., 2015; Clancy, 1996; Gonzalez-Escobedo et al., 2011; Gradmann, 2010; Yokchoo et al., 2019) |
| Variable Contact Rates | | Contact rates that affect the reactions of pandemics are accounted for | (Brauer, 2011; Esteva & Vargas, 1999; Greenhalgh & Das, 1995) |
| SIR with Diffusion | | Spatiotemporal populations describing the densities and time patterns of S, I, R individuals | (Bekiros & Kouloumpou, 2020; Fuentes & Kuperman, 1999; Schurz & Tosun, 2015) |
| SIR Model on Networks | | More realistic model with non-homogeneous population into consideration | (Boccara et al., 1992; Chang et al., 2019; Dottori & Fabricius, 2015; Eames & Keeling, 2002; Huang et al., 2016; Li & Yousef, 2019; Lindquist et al., 2011; Stolerman et al., 2015; Yan et al., 2018) |

| Model | Variables | Specifics | References |
|---|---|---|---|
| SIRS | Susceptible -> Infectious -> Recovered -> Susceptible | Models consider Individuals who Recover however with no immunity hence they are prone to disease Susceptibility | (Adda & Bichara, 2011; Cai et al., 2017; Chalub & Souza, 2011; Corberán-Vallet & Santonja, 2014; Dolgoarshinnykh & Lalley, 2003; Li et al., 2017; Paladini et al., 2011; Rao et al., 2019; Wang, 2015; Zhao et al., 2014) |

Numerous examples of SIR models for various disease spread mechanism can be found (Angstmann et al., 2016; Dike et al., 2017, 2018; Guo et al., 2006; Sanz et al., 2014; Takeuchi et al., 2000). Blackwood and Child (2018) is a paper for budding modelers in infectious modeling (Blackwood & Childs, 2018). The importance of the compartmental modelling and their significance in the epidemic modelling was reviewed by Tolles & Luong (2020) (Tolles & Luong, 2020). Apart from the models reviewed in this chapter, numerous other models developed are available in the literature. A model with quarantine species follows susceptible, exposed, infected and quarantine pattern (Chen et al., 2017; Xia et al., 2018). Anguelov (2013) describes a model which is a hybrid between the SIR and SEIR models (Anguelov et al., 2013). Modified SEIR model with a vaccination species termed as SVEIR for tuberculosis was also developed and analyzed (Adebimpe et al., 2020; Cai & Li, 2009; Gao & Huang, 2018; Sahu & Dhar, 2012; Zhou & Cui, 2011); Widyaningsih et al., (2019) details on the MSVIR models for Tetanus disease (Widyaningsih et al., 2019).

In addition to the mechanistic SIR models in observing the trends of infectious disease modelling other Statistical and Empirical based surveillance approaches have also been proposed. Among which Empirical AI and ML based approaches are being attracting focus in recent years. Artificial intelligence and analysis have been identified as a prominent tool in the analysis of such big data acquired from the experimental analysis. Several tools have been developed in the field of AI in the analysis of OMICS data. Some of the include Bayesian networks, Artificial Neural Networks, Fuzzy Clustering, Support Vector Machine, Artificial Immune System, ARIMA, Random Forest, Decision Tree, K- Neighbouring, unsupervised learning etc. (Mohamadou et al., 2020; Park et al., 2021; Philemon et al., 2019; Surya, 2018; Taylor et al., 2018). Further the use of AI and ML in Disease Modelling was detailed by Agrebi and Larbi in their book chapter (Agrebi & Larbi, 2020).These tools have been observed to be part of the analysis of diseases in terms of their diagnosis, outbreak, source of infection, pandemic, epidemic, resistance prediction, drug discovery, therapies, host pathogen interactions etc,. Thus results in several positive outcomes like decision support, saving cost, time, life, enabling low income countries, personalized medicine, forensic approach etc.

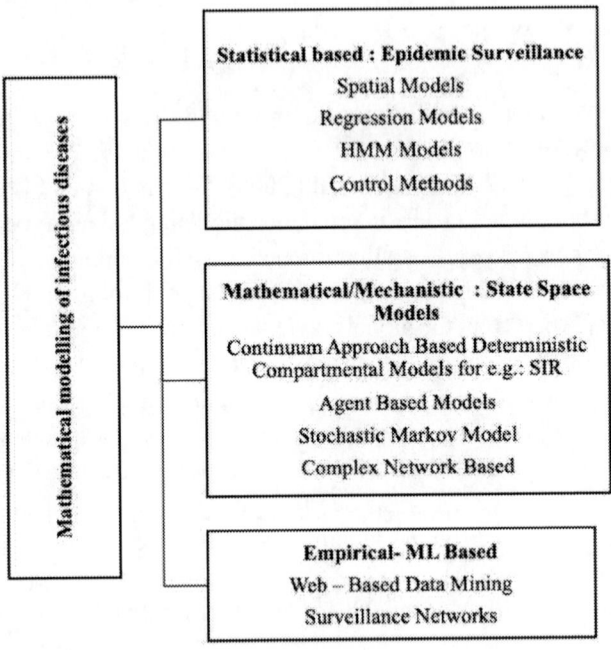

**Figure 3.** Simple classification of various different types of mathematical models utilized for modelling and analysis of epidemics.

Mechanistic model for diseases might be more useful. There are very few mechanical models available for infectious diseases. Individual based models (IBM) are less frequently utilized comparing to compartmental models. It is a bottom-up modeling strategy which allows for history of every individual to be tracked and network structures to be explicitly represented (Willem et al., 2017). Gambhir et al., (2015) summarizes on the methods to model the novel influenza virus, related questions to be asked before modelling, data requirements for modelling depending on the type of model chosen (Gambhir et al., 2015). The dynamics of spread depends on the underlying host contact network. Therefore, the social network-based graph theoretical models are utilized to track the disease spread within communities and across community.

Here the individuals within community are the nodes and the interaction between them leads to disease spread which is represented as edge. Comparing to transitional compartmental models, such graph theory-based social or community network models for disease spread are relatively recent (Keeling and Eames, 2005). In recent literature there are numerous such integrated model combining SIR model on Networks are available (Chang et al., 2019; Eames & Keeling, 2002; Maheshwari & Albert, 2020; Salathé & Jones, 2010). These models account for the practical heterogenous contact structure and spread among and within community (refer Figure 2). Different modelling methods are grouped and shown in Figure 3. Some examples of diverse modelling and simulation tools are summarised in Table 2.

**Table 2.** Modeling tools for epidemic simulations

| Computational Tool | Function | Reference |
|---|---|---|
| GLEaMviz | Models' global epidemic and travel | (Broeck et al., 2011) http://www.gleamviz.org/ |
| epiDMS | Epidemic simulation data management system | (Liu et al., 2016) |
| Opensource Modeling tools | Modeling tools assembled by Institute of Disease Biology (IDB) | https://www.idmod.org/tools |
| Epigrass | Facilitates comprehensive spatiotemporal simulations particularly for large scale models Enables visualizing the geographic information system and stores the results in GIS format | (Coelho et al., 2008) |
| Jena Adaptable Modelling Systems (JAMS) | Open-source software and is structured in modules that are reusable in new models | (Falenski et al., 2013) |
| Netlogo | Agent Based Modelling tool Consists of programming languages along with graphical tools for constructing interfaces. Provides Environment for modelling complex natural and social phenomenon | (Berryman & Angus, 2010) |
| EMULSION | AI based stochastic epidemiological modeling tool for various systems including human, animals and plants | (Picault et al., 2019) |
| EpiModel | open source, R package, used to study of population dynamics for disease transmission by building simulating and analysing of mathematical models | (Jenness et al., 2018) |

**Table 2.** (Continued)

| Computational Tool | Function | Reference |
|---|---|---|
| EMOD(Epidemiological MODeling Software) | An agent-based model developed by IDM to advance the understanding of disease dynamics | (Bershteyn et al., 2018) https://docs.idmod.org/projects/emod-generic/en/latest/model-sir.html |
| Eon (Epidemics on networks) | python package for the analysis of networks based on SIS and SIR models | (Miller & Ting, 2019) |
| Epydemic | package built on python networkx package for network modelling of SIS and SIR epidemic models | (Dobson, 2017) |
| AceMod | agent based modelling framework for influenza in Australia | (Cliff et al., 2018) |

## 4. Examples/Case Studies

Lessons from the previously developed epidemiological models may serve as primer for learning the essential skills and gaining expertise in epidemiological modeling (Willem et al., 2017). Outcomes of various models are analyzed to explore reliable predictions and assess the robustness of the model (Huppert & Katriel, 2013).

### 4.1. COVID-19

The spread of COVID-19 has posed several new challenges to the society and scientists across globe. Network model of human- human interaction proposed by Maheshwari and Albert (2020) for COVID-19 considers the individuals to be represented by nodes and the edges represents various interactions including family, workplace, essential needs and social interactions (Maheshwari & Albert, 2020). Each of the individuals are considered to be at one of the following four states, namely susceptible, infected, immune, and dead. This model based on the available data and parameters simulated spread of the infection in presence of various mitigation scenarios including lockdown and emergence of second wave (Maheshwari & Albert, 2020). Similar network-based model has illustrated the presence of super-spreaders in Romanian population. The skewed distribution of the out-degree score of the network allowed to infer that COVID-19 patients transmitted the virus in different rates (Hâncean et al., 2020). A network model embedded with SIR model (Network augmented SIR/ NSIR) developed has introduced uncertainty and path dependence associated with network unlike uniform mixing assumption of SIR models. This model has predicted the effectiveness of various social distancing strategies in flattening the spread and they have also observed that the epidemic dynamics are sensitive to policy timing and duration (Karaivanov, 2020).

During the beginning of the pandemic apart from SIR and modified SIR models such simplistic network-based approaches provided insights on emergence of disease pattern, infection spread, super-spreaders, effect of mitigation strategies etc. Later with availability of data, complexity of the models has also increased. And mitigation strategy such as vaccination and effect of heard immunity were included in the models. There are systematic reviews that consolidates various models available for COVID-19 (Shakeel et al., 2021). There are also comparative studies on the different types of modeling and their prediction abilities (Abolmaali & Shirzaei, 2021). As guidance towards mechanistic modeling of the COVID19 pandemic a community driven open access effort has led to the development of the detailed disease map referred as C19DMap (Ostaszewski et al., 2021). This effort has provided new testable hypothesis and disease signature for mechanistic modelling and systems biology research community.

## 4.2. Influenza

Extensive epidemiological studies on influenza is required to explore scientific strategies for its prevention (Chen et al., 2020). Quiroette and team (2020) modelled the spatial infection pattern of Influenza A Virus (IAV) by constructing partial differential equations (PDEs) for the two spatial parameters diffusion and advection (Quirouette et al., 2020). Infection is localized within the human respiratory tract (HRT) considering the diffusion through periciliary fluid (PCF) and advection effectively sweeping away the IAV. The concentration of the virus in the spatial model depends on depth along with time consequently it also depicts that the infections is faster in the upper HRT (Quirouette et al., 2020). Gradually, these strains of influenza attain changes and become resistant which is deadly. A two- strain (Resistant and non-resistant) four compartment model constructed exhibits the co-existence of the two- strains along with their difference in the mode of transmission. Saturated, bilinear incident rates were attributed for the resistant non- resistant strains where it was seen that the resistant strains rapidly seize due to the reduced virulence from the mutations (Baba et al., 2021).

Modeling the transmission of the global outbreak strain H1N1 (Swine flu 2009) has predicted the evolution of disease in the Morocco province. A simple SIR model given by non-linear differential equations predicting the disease to be endemic when the reproduction number is more than one. Numerical simulations illustrated the evolution as a time period from the point of disease reaching maximum till it decreasing down to an endemic equilibrium state (Hattaf & Yousfi, 2009). Along with swine flu (H1N1), the other strains of influenza include avian (H5N1) and the seasonal influenza (H3N1). The seasonal influenza among them usually doesn't cause death therefore the seasonal influenza SIR model considers the population constant. The transmission or spreading can be checked from the minimum value of p given by the reproduction number (R0). The simulation of the model using parameters from the previous research gives the proportion of people taking treatment (Kharis & Arifudin, 2017). Further improvements of such mathematical models on influenza will provide better predictions on the transmission and the treatment conditions.

### 4.3. Ebola Virus Disease (EVD)

The necessity to eradicate the Ebola virus disease has emphasized the need to understand the features of the epidemics with its transmission dynamics and to evaluate the containment measures (Dike et al., 2018). There are six species of Ebola virus out of which four causes the disease in humans. To assess the spread dynamics of these viruses through direct or indirect transmission a SEIR model was constructed. The model addresses the gaps in mathematical analysis of the previous compartmental SEIR model. Disease free equilibrium, Endemic equilibrium are the two equilibrium points considered for the model. The numerical interpretations were solved using both Runge-Kutta ($RK_4$) and non-standard finite difference (NSFD) scheme showing that NSFD is more reliable in preserving the nonnegativity and boundedness of the solutions. Graph presented from the analysis gives the dynamics of the disease (Rafiq et al., 2020). Generally, in the case of dynamics when $R_0$ is greater than one it is expected for the epidemic to infect a significant percentage of the population. The $R_0$ value obtained from the previous fitting compartmental models for Ebola was found to be between 1.34 and 3.65. The effective reproductive ratio ($R_t$) reduces under medical or social response and the heterogeneity can cause an outbreak to become extinct even when $R_t$ is greater (House, 2014). Considering the quarantine state, where the individuals associated with Ebola infected, or Ebola deceased humans are sorted and quarantined. The population is divided into 11 states representing the model variables and the non-quarantined population among them are also included in the model. Overall, the model depicts that quarantine, acting as a buffer zone, is not completely sufficient to eradicate the disease however reduces the daily infection rate(Ngwa & Teboh-Ewungkem, 2016).Insights on the effectiveness of these control strategies can be observed from the models providing possible further recommendations on them.

## 4.4. Zika

Zika virus was neglected for many years until the major outbreak occurred (2007) (Wiratsudakul et al., 2018). It is closely related to the dengue viruses. Compartmental, spatial, meta population, network and individual- based are the model architectures used in studying the Zika epidemic. In the development of these complex modelling framework, preparing them prior to outbreak is much needed which includes the future Zika epidemic preparation (Wiratsudakul et al., 2018). A deterministic SEIR model proposed by Gao et al. is used in studying the Zika virus spread dynamics between humans and mosquitoes (Gao et al., 2016). The models constructed are also based on these modes of transmission such as horizontal transmission, vertical transmission and the one combining both the modes (Bessey et al., 2019). Control measures to prevent the transmission is the major goal in disease epidemiology where the control theory and the possible elimination are presented from the numerical results of the described model. Model proposed by E.O Alzahrani considers the mutant Zika virus in presence of three controls which includes bed nets, spraying insecticides and treatment efforts. Analysis shows that the mentioned set of controls are very effective for the human infection elimination in the society (Alzahrani et al., 2021). Thus, the models also propose effective control strategies for controlling the spread of Zika.

## 5. Model Analysis and Prediction Tools

During the course of modeling and analysis of disease progression, various computational and mathematical modeling tools were also developed. Some of these simulation tools considers the critical determinants of disease spread mechanism such as demography, population distribution, sub population level effects, morbidity and mortality, travel, and migration, etc.

GLEaMviz is a computational tool to simulate realistic epidemic scenarios (Broeck et al., 2011). Table 2 provides some of the large-scale simulation tools that considers various crucial factors such as travel, economics, health care systems, vaccination, and control strategies etc. at larger scale during epidemic. Some of these are publicly available for simulation and analysis explorations. Heslop et al., (2017) review twenty such freely available tools more elaborately. Institute of Disease Biology has consolidated some of the useful modeling, analysis, computational and visualizations tools for exploration (Heslop et al., 2017). These are opensource tools and freely available for scientific community. Caprelli et al., 2014 reviews the tools for pandemic modelling that are based on R and Python tools (Caprarelli & Fletcher, 2014).

## Conclusion

There are numerous challenges involved in collecting data and finding the right parameters for predictions, yet the models are futuristic tools that provide additional insights into the disease spread mechanism. Such insights can assist in the process of challenging scientific questions on emergence of disease, shift in the dynamic spread, effectiveness of the controlling strategies and policy decisions. Molecular mechanism of host, pathogen integrated models may provide additional mechanics understanding of disease progression, management, and treatment strategy.

## References

Abolmaali, S., & Shirzaei, S. (2021). Forecasting COVID-19 Number of Cases by Implementing ARIMA and SARIMA with Grid Search in the United States. *medRxiv*.

Adda, P., & Bichara, D. J. (2011). Global stability for SIR and SIRS models with differential mortality. *International Journal of Pure and Applied Mathematics, 80.* https://doi.org/https://doi.org/10.48550/arXiv.1112.2662.

Adebimpe, O., Abiodun, O., Oludoun, O., & Gbadamosi, B. (2020). Analysis of an SEIV Epidemic Model with Temporary Immunity and Saturated Incidence Rate. *2020 International Conference in Mathematics, Computer Engineering and Computer Science (ICMCECS).*

Agrebi, S., & Larbi, A. (2020). Use of artificial intelligence in infectious diseases. In *Artificial intelligence in precision health* (pp. 415-438). Elsevier.

Al-Raeei, M. (2020). The forecasting of COVID-19 with mortality using SIRD epidemic model for the United States, Russia, China, and the Syrian Arab Republic. *AIP Advances, 10*(6), 065325. https://doi.org/10.1063/5.0014275.

Allen, L. J. S. J. M. b. (1994). Some discrete-time SI, SIR, and SIS epidemic models. *Mathematical Biosciences, 124*(1), 83-105.

Almeida, R., Brito Da Cruz, A. M. C., Martins, N., & Monteiro, M. T. T. (2019). An epidemiological MSEIR model described by the Caputo fractional derivative. *International Journal of Dynamics and Control, 7*(2), 776-784. https://doi.org/10.1007/s40435-018-0492-1.

Alzahrani, E. O., Ahmad, W., Khan, M. A., & Malebary, S. J. (2021). Optimal control strategies of Zika virus model with mutant. *Communications in Nonlinear Science and Numerical Simulation, 93,* 105532.

Ameen, I., Baleanu, D., & Ali, H. M. (2020). An efficient algorithm for solving the fractional optimal control of SIRV epidemic model with a combination of vaccination and treatment. *Chaos, Solitons & Fractals, 137,* 109892. https://doi.org/10.1016/j.chaos.2020.109892.

Amira; Torres, R. (2018). Analysis, simulation and optimal control of a seir model for ebola virus with demographic effects. *Communications Faculty Of Science University of Ankara Series A1Mathematics and Statistics, 67*(1), 179-197. https://doi.org/10.1501/commua1_0000000841.

Andrade, J., & Duggan, J. J. E. (2020). An evaluation of Hamiltonian Monte Carlo performance to calibrate age-structured compartmental SEIR models to incidence data. *Epidemics, 33,* 100415.

Angstmann, C. N., Henry, B. I., & McGann, A. V. (2016). A Fractional Order Recovery SIR Model from a Stochastic Process. *Bull Math Biol, 78*(3), 468-499. https://doi.org/10.1007/s11538-016-0151-7.

Anguelov, R., Dumont, Y., Lubuma, J., & Mureithi, E. (2013). Stability Analysis and Dynamics Preserving Nonstandard Finite Difference Schemes for a Malaria Model. *Mathematical Population Studies, 20*(2), 101-122. https://doi.org/10.1080/08898480.2013.777240.

Anguelov, R., Dumont, Y., Lubuma, J., Shillor, M., Simos, T. E., Psihoyios, G., & Tsitouras, Ch. (2009). Comparison of some standard and nonstandard numerical methods for the mseir epidemiological model. *AIP Conference Proceedings,* 1209–1212.

Apenteng, O. O., & Ismail, N. A. (2014). The Impact of the Wavelet Propagation Distribution on SEIRS Modeling with Delay. *PLoS ONE, 9*(6), e98288. https://doi.org/10.1371/journal.pone.0098288.

Arachchi, D. K. M., & Hasanthika, N. H. E. Stochasticity in SIRV Models with Vaccination and Reversion for the Transmission of Epidemic diseases. *Conference: International Forum for Mathematical Modeling.*

Arif, M. S., Raza, A., Rafiq, M., & Bibi, M. (2019). A reliable numerical analysis for stochastic hepatitis B virus epidemic model with the migration effect. *Iranian Journal of Science and Technology, Transactions A: Science, 43*(5), 2477-2492.

Baba, I. A., Ahmad, H., Alsulami, M., Abualnaja, K. M., & Altanji, M. (2021). A mathematical model to study resistance and non-resistance strains of influenza. *Results in Physics, 26,* 104390.

Balzotti, C., D'Ovidio, M., & Loreti, P. (2020). Fractional SIS Epidemic Models. *Fractal and Fractional, 4*(3), 44. https://doi.org/10.3390/fractalfract4030044.

Bekiros, S., & Kouloumpou, D. (2020). SBDiEM: A new mathematical model of infectious disease dynamics. *Chaos, Solitons & Fractals, 136,* 109828. https://doi.org/10.1016/j.chaos.2020.109828.

Berger, D. W., Herkenhoff, K. F., & Mongey, S. (2020). An seir infectious disease model with testing and conditional quarantine. *SSRN Electronic Journal.*

Berryman, M. J., & Angus, S. D. (2010). Tutorials on agent-based modelling with NetLogo and network analysis with Pajek. In *Complex Physical, Biophysical and Econophysical systems* (pp. 351-375). World Scientific.

Bershteyn, A., Gerardin, J., Bridenbecker, D., Lorton, C. W., Bloedow, J., Baker, R. S., Wiswell, C. N. (2018). Implementation and applications of EMOD, an individual-based multi-disease modeling platform. *Pathogens and Disease, 76*(5). https://doi.org/10.1093/femspd/fty059.

Bessey, K., Mavis, M., Rebaza, J., & Zhang, J. (2019). Global stability analysis of a general model of Zika virus. *Nonautonomous Dynamical Systems, 6*(1), 18-34.

Bichara, D., Iggidr, A., & Sallet, G. (2014). Global analysis of multi-strains SIS, SIR and MSIR epidemic models. *Journal of Applied Mathematics and Computing, 44*(1-2), 273-292. https://doi.org/10.1007/s12190-013-0693-x.

Bichara, D., Kang, Y., Castillo-Chavez, C., Horan, R., & Perrings, C. (2015). SIS and SIR Epidemic Models Under Virtual Dispersal. *Bulletin of Mathematical Biology, 77*(11), 2004-2034. https://doi.org/10.1007/s11538-015-0113-5.

Biswas, M. H. A., Paiva, L. T., & De Pinho, M. D. R. (2014). A SEIR model for control of infectious diseases with constraints. *J. Mathematical Biosciences and Engineering., 11*(4), 761. https://doi.org/10.3934/mbe.2014.11.761.

Bjørnstad, O. N., Shea, K., Krzywinski, M., & Altman, N. (2020). The SEIRS model for infectious disease dynamics. *Nature Methods, 17*(6), 557-558. https://doi.org/10.1038/s41592-020-0856-2.

Blackwood, J. C., & Childs, L. M. (2018). An introduction to compartmental modeling for the budding infectious disease modeler. *Letters in Biomathematics, 5*(1), 195-221. https://doi.org/10.1080/23737867.2018.1509026.

Blaizot, S., Herzog, S. A., Abrams, S., Theeten, H., Litzroth, A., & Hens, N. (2019). Sample size calculation for estimating key epidemiological parameters using serological data

and mathematical modelling. *BMC Medical Research Methodology*, *19*(1). https://doi.org/10.1186/s12874-019-0692-1.
Boccara, N., Cheong, K. J. J. o. P. A. M., & General. (1992). Automata network SIR models for the spread of infectious diseases in populations of moving individuals. *Journal of Physics A: Mathematical and General*, *25*(9), 2447.
Brauer, F. (2011). Variable infectivity in communicable disease models. *World Congress of Nonlinear Analysts' 92*.
Broeck, W. V. D., Gioannini, C., Gonçalves, B., Quaggiotto, M., Colizza, V., & Vespignani, A. (2011). The GLEaMviz computational tool, a publicly available software to explore realistic epidemic spreading scenarios at the global scale. *BMC Infectious Diseases*, *11*(1), 37. https://doi.org/10.1186/1471-2334-11-37.
Bronsvoort, B. M. D., Handel, I. G., Nfon, C. K., Sørensen, K.-J., Malirat, V., Bergmann, I., ... Morgan, K. L. (2016). Redefining the "carrier" state for foot-and-mouth disease from the dynamics of virus persistence in endemically affected cattle populations. *Scientific Reports*, *6*(1), 29059. https://doi.org/10.1038/srep29059.
Cador, C., Rose, N., Willem, L., & Andraud, M. (2016). Maternally derived immunity extends swine influenza A virus persistence within farrow-to-finish pig farms: insights from a stochastic event-driven metapopulation model. *PloS One*, *11*(9), e0163672.
Cai, L.-M., & Li, X.-Z. (2009). Analysis of a SEIV epidemic model with a nonlinear incidence rate. *Applied Mathematical Modelling*, *33*(7), 2919-2926.
Cai, Y., Kang, Y., & Wang, W. (2017). A stochastic SIRS epidemic model with nonlinear incidence rate. *Applied Mathematics and Computation*, *305*, 221-240. https://doi.org/10.1016/j.amc.2017.02.003.
Cao, J., Wang, Y., Alofi, A., Al-Mazrooei, A., & Elaiw, A. (2015). Global stability of an epidemic model with carrier state in heterogeneous networks. *IMA Journal of Applied Mathematics*, *80*(4), 1025-1048. https://doi.org/10.1093/imamat/hxu040.
Capistrán, M. A., Christen, J. A., & Velasco-Hernández, J. X. (2012). Towards uncertainty quantification and inference in the stochastic SIR epidemic model. *Mathematical Biosciences*, *240*(2), 250-259. https://doi.org/10.1016/j.mbs.2012.08.005.
Caprarelli, G., & Fletcher, S. (2014). A brief review of spatial analysis concepts and tools used for mapping, containment and risk modelling of infectious diseases and other illnesses. *Parasitology*, *141*(5), 581-601.
Castillo-Chavez, C., Blower, S., Van den Driessche, P., Kirschner, D., & Yakubu, A.-A. (2002). *Mathematical Approaches for Emerging and Reemerging Infectious Diseases: Models, Methods, and Theory* (Vol. 126). Springer Science & Business Media.
Cevik, M., Tate, M., Lloyd, O., Maraolo, A. E., Schafers, J., & Ho, A. (2021). SARS-CoV-2, SARS-CoV, and MERS-CoV viral load dynamics, duration of viral shedding, and infectiousness: a systematic review and meta-analysis. *The Lancet Microbe*, *2*(1), e13-e22.
Chalub, F. A. C. C., & Souza, M. O. (2011). The SIR epidemic model from a PDE point of view. *Mathematical and Computer Modelling*, *53*(7-8), 1568-1574. https://doi.org/10.1016/j.mcm.2010.05.036.
Chang, S. L., Piraveenan, M., & Prokopenko, M. (2019). The Effects of Imitation Dynamics on Vaccination Behaviours in SIR-Network Model. *International Journal of*

*Environmental Research and Public Health*, *16*(14), 2477. https://doi.org/10.3390/ijerph16142477.

Chen, D. (2020). On the Integrability of the SIR Epidemic Model with Vital Dynamics. *Advances in Mathematical Physics*, *2020*, 1-10. https://doi.org/10.1155/2020/5869275.

Chen, X., Cao, J., Park, J. H., & Qiu, J. (2017). Stability analysis and estimation of domain of attraction for the endemic equilibrium of an SEIQ epidemic model. *Nonlinear Dynamics*, *87*(2), 975-985. https://doi.org/10.1007/s11071-016-3092-7.

Chen, Y., Leng, K., Lu, Y., Wen, L., Qi, Y., Gao, W., . . . Sun, B. (2020). Epidemiological features and time-series analysis of influenza incidence in urban and rural areas of Shenyang, China, 2010–2018. *Epidemiology & Infection*, *148*.

Clancy, D. (1996). Carrier-borne epidemic models incorporating population mobility. *Math Biosci*, *132*(2), 185-204. https://doi.org/10.1016/0025-5564(95)00063-1.

Cliff, O. M., Harding, N., Piraveenan, M., Erten, E. Y., Gambhir, M., & Prokopenko, M. (2018). Investigating spatiotemporal dynamics and synchrony of influenza epidemics in Australia: An agent-based modelling approach. *Simulation Modelling Practice and Theory*, *87*, 412-431. https://doi.org/10.1016/j.simpat.2018.07.005.

Coelho, F. C., Cruz, O. G., & Codeço, C. T. (2008). Epigrass: a tool to study disease spread in complex networks. *Source Code for Biology and Medicine*, *3*(1), 1-9.

Cooke, K. L., & van den Driessche, P. (1996). Analysis of an SEIRS epidemic model with two delays. *J Math Biol*, *35*(2), 240-260. https://doi.org/10.1007/s002850050051.

Corberán-Vallet, A., & Santonja, F. J. (2014). A Bayesian SIRS model for the analysis of respiratory syncytial virus in the region of Valencia, Spain. *Biom J*, *56*(5), 808-818. https://doi.org/10.1002/bimj.201300194.

Denphedtnong, A., Chinviriyasit, S., & Chinviriyasit, W. (2013). On the dynamics of SEIRS epidemic model with transport-related infection. *Mathematical Biosciences*, *245*(2), 188-205. https://doi.org/10.1016/j.mbs.2013.07.001.

Despommier, D. D., & Karapelou, J. W. (2012). *Parasite Life Cycles*. Springer Science & Business Media.

Dike, C. O., Zainuddin, Z. M., & Dike, I. J. (2017). Susceptible Infected Removed Epidemic Model Extension for Efficient Analysis of Ebola Virus Disease Transmission. *J. Advanced Science Letters*, *23*(9), 9107-9114.

Dike, C. O., Zainuddin, Z. M., & Dike, I. J. (2018). Mathematical Models for Mitigating Ebola Virus Disease Transmission: A Review. *Advanced Science Letters*, *24*(5), 3536-3543.

Dobson, S. (2017). Epydemic: Epidemic simulations on networks in Python. https://pyepydemic.readthedocs.io/en/latest/index.html.

Dolgoarshinnykh, R. G., & Lalley, S. P. (2003). *Epidemic Modelling: SIRS Models* University of Chicago, Department of Statistics].

Dottori, M., & Fabricius, G. J. (2015). SIR model on a dynamical network and the endemic state of an infectious disease. *Physica A: Statistical Mechanics and its Applications*, *434*, 25-35. https://doi.org/https://doi.org/10.1016/j.physa.2015.04.007.

Dukic, V., Lopes, H. F., & Polson, N. G. (2012). Tracking Epidemics With Google Flu Trends Data and a State-Space SEIR Model. *Journal of the American Statistical Association*, *107*(500), 1410-1426. https://doi.org/10.1080/01621459.2012.713876.

Eames, K. T. D., & Keeling, M. J. (2002). Modeling dynamic and network heterogeneities in the spread of sexually transmitted diseases. *Proceedings of the National Academy of Sciences, 99*(20), 13330-13335. https://doi.org/10.1073/pnas.202244299.

Esteva, L., & Vargas, C. (1999). A model for dengue disease with variable human population. *Journal of Mathematical Biology, 38*(3), 220-240. https://doi.org/10.1007/s002850050147.

Fajar, R. J. G. (2019). Stability Analysis and Computer Simulation of MSIR Mathematics Model to Prevent Hepatitis B Virus Spread by Vaccination. *Gut & Liver.* 13 (6), p. 104-104.

Falenski, A., Filter, M., Thöns, C., Weiser, A. A., Wigger, J.-F., Davis, M., . . . Kaufman, J. H. (2013). A generic open-source software framework supporting scenario simulations in bioterrorist crises. *Biosecurity and Bioterrorism: Biodefense Strategy, Practice, and Science, 11*(S1), S134-S145.

Fan, M., Li, M. Y., & Wang, K. (2001). Global stability of an SEIS epidemic model with recruitment and a varying total population size. *Math Biosci, 170*(2), 199-208. https://doi.org/10.1016/s0025-5564(00)00067-5.

Fuentes, M. A., & Kuperman, M. N. (1999). Cellular automata and epidemiological models with spatial dependence. *Physica A Statistical Mechanics and its Applications, 267*(3-4), 471-486. https://doi.org/10.1016/S0378-4371(99)00027-8.

Gambhir, M., Bozio, C., O'Hagan, J. J., Uzicanin, A., Johnson, L. E., Biggerstaff, M., & Swerdlow, D. L. (2015). Infectious Disease Modeling Methods as Tools for Informing Response to Novel Influenza Viruses of Unknown Pandemic Potential. *Clinical Infectious Diseases, 60* (suppl_1), S11-S19. https://doi.org/10.1093/cid/civ083.

Gao, D., Lou, Y., He, D., Porco, T. C., Kuang, Y., Chowell, G., & Ruan, S. (2016). Prevention and control of Zika as a mosquito-borne and sexually transmitted disease: a mathematical modeling analysis. *Scientific Reports, 6*(1), 1-10.

Gao, D.-P., & Huang, N.-J. (2018). Optimal control analysis of a tuberculosis model. *Applied Mathematical Modelling, 58*, 47-64. https://doi.org/10.1016/j.apm.2017.12.027.

Gao, S., Chen, L., & Teng, Z. (2007). Impulsive vaccination of an SEIRS model with time delay and varying total population size. *Bull Math Biol, 69*(2), 731-745. https://doi.org/10.1007/s11538-006-9149-x.

Gbolahan, B. (2010). A Deterministic Mathematical Model of Measles in Newborn(s) Using the MSEIR Endemic Model. *Nigerian Journal of Mathematics and Applications,* Vol. 20, pg. 75-81.

Getz, W. M., Salter, R., & Mgbara, W. (2019). Adequacy of SEIR models when epidemics have spatial structure: Ebola in Sierra Leone. *Philosophical Transactions of the Royal Society B: Biological Sciences, 374*(1775), 20180282. https://doi.org/10.1098/rstb.2018.0282.

Giubilei, R. (2020). Closed form solution of the SIR model for the COVID-19 outbreak in Italy. *J. MedRxiv.* https://doi.org/10.1101/2020.06.06.20124313.

Gonzalez-Escobedo, G., Marshall, J. M., & Gunn, J. S. (2011). Chronic and acute infection of the gall bladder by Salmonella Typhi: understanding the carrier state. *Nature Reviews Microbiology, 9*(1), 9-14. https://doi.org/10.1038/nrmicro2490.

Gradmann, C. (2010). Robert Koch and the invention of the carrier state: tropical medicine, veterinary infections and epidemiology around 1900. *Stud Hist Philos Biol Biomed Sci, 41*(3), 232-240. https://doi.org/10.1016/j.shpsc.2010.04.012.

Grassly, N. C., & Fraser, C. (2008). Mathematical models of infectious disease transmission. *Nature Reviews Microbiology, 6*(6), 477-487. https://doi.org/10.1038/nrmicro1845.

Greenhalgh, D. (1997). Hopf bifurcation in epidemic models with a latent period and nonpermanent immunity. *Mathematical and Computer Modelling, 25*(2), 85-107.

Greenhalgh, D., & Das, R. (1995). Modeling epidemics with variable contact rates. *J. Theoretical Population Biology, 47*(2), 129-179. https://doi.org/10.1006/tpbi.1995.1006.

Guo, H., Li, M. Y., & Shuai, Z. (2006). Global stability of the endemic equilibrium of multigroup SIR epidemic models. *Canadian Applied Mathematics Quarterly 14*(3), 259-284.

Guo, S.-M., Li, X.-Z., & Song, X.-Y. (2010). Stability of an age-structured SEIS epidemic model with infectivity in incubative period. *International Journal of Biomathematics, 3*(03), 299-312.

Hâncean, M.-G., Perc, M., & Lerner, J. (2020). Early spread of COVID-19 in Romania: imported cases from Italy and human-to-human transmission networks. *Royal Society Open Science, 7*(7), 200780.

Harko, T., & Mak, M. K. (2020). Series solution of the Susceptible-Infected-Recovered (SIR) epidemic model with vital dynamics via the Adomian and Laplace-Adomian Decomposition Methods. *arXiv:2009.00434 [q-bio.PE]*.

Hattaf, K., & Yousfi, N. (2009). Mathematical model of the influenza A (H1N1) infection. *Advanced Studies in Biology, 1*(8), 383-390.

Heslop, D. J., Chughtai, A. A., Bui, C. M., & MacIntyre, C. R. (2017). Publicly available software tools for decision-makers during an emergent epidemic—Systematic evaluation of utility and usability. *Epidemics, 21*, 1-12.

Hethcote, H. W. (1978). An immunization model for a heterogeneous population. *Theoretical Population Biology, 14*(3), 338-349.

Hethcote, H. W. (2000). The mathematics of infectious diseases. *SIAM Review, 42*(4), 599-653.

Hethcote, H. W. (2009). Epidemiology models with variable population size. In *Mathematical Understanding of Infectious Disease Dynamics* (pp. 63-89). World Scientific.

Hethcote, H. W., & van den Driessche, P. (1995). An SIS epidemic model with variable population size and a delay. *J Math Biol, 34*(2), 177-194. https://doi.org/10.1007/BF00178772.

Hethcote, H. W., & Van Den Driessche, P. (2000). Two SIS epidemiologic models with delays. *Journal of Mathematical Biology, 40*(1), 3-26. https://doi.org/10.1007/s002850050003.

Hill, A. N., & Longini, I. M., Jr. (2003). The critical vaccination fraction for heterogeneous epidemic models. *Math Biosci, 181*(1), 85-106. https://doi.org/10.1016/s0025-5564(02)00129-3.

House, T. (2014). Epidemiological dynamics of Ebola outbreaks. *Elife, 3*, e03908.

Huang, C., Cao, J., Wen, F., & Yang, X. (2016). Stability Analysis of SIR Model with Distributed Delay on Complex Networks. *PLOS ONE, 11*(8), e0158813. https://doi.org/10.1371/journal.pone.0158813.

Huppert, A., & Katriel, G. (2013). Mathematical modelling and prediction in infectious disease epidemiology. *Clinical Microbiology and Infection, 19*(11), 999-1005.

Inaba, H. (2006). Age-structured homogeneous epidemic systems with application to the MSEIR epidemic model. *Journal of Mathematical Biology, 54*(1), 101-146. https://doi.org/10.1007/s00285-006-0033-y.

Ishikawa, M. (2018). Mathematical Analysis of the Stochastic Delayed Epidemic Models with Reinfection. *Proceedings of the ISCIE International Symposium on Stochastic Systems Theory and its Applications, 2018*(0), 147-152. https://doi.org/10.5687/sss.2018.147.

Jenness, S. M., Goodreau, S. M., & Morris, M. (2018). EpiModel: An R Package for Mathematical Modeling of Infectious Disease over Networks. *J Stat Softw, 84*. https://doi.org/10.18637/jss.v084.i08.

Jia, J., & Xiao, J. (2018). Stability analysis of a disease resistance SEIRS model with nonlinear incidence rate. *Advances in Difference Equations, 2018*(1). https://doi.org/10.1186/s13662-018-1494-1.

Jiang, Z., Ma, W., & Wei, J. (2016). Global Hopf bifurcation and permanence of a delayed SEIRS epidemic model. *Mathematics and Computers in Simulation, 122*, 35-54.

Jiao, J., Chen, L., & Cai, S. (2008). An SEIRS epidemic model with two delays and pulse vaccination. *Journal of Systems Science and Complexity, 21*(2), 217-225. https://doi.org/10.1007/s11424-008-9105-y.

Karaivanov, A. (2020). A social network model of COVID-19. *Plos One, 15*(10), e0240878.

Kermack, W. O., & McKendrick, A. G. (1927). A contribution to the mathematical theory of epidemics. *Proceedings of the Royal Society of London, 115*(772), 700-721.

Kharis, M., & Arifudin, R. (2017). Mathematical model of seasonal influenza with treatment in constant population. *Journal of Physics: Conference Series.*

Kutrolli, G., Kutrolli, M., & Meco, E. (2020). The Origin, Diffusion and the Comparison of Ode Numerical Solutions Used by SIR Model in Order to Predict SARS-CoV-2 in Nordic Countries. *International Journal of Medical and Health Sciences, 15*, 33-62.

Kuznetsov, Y. A., & Piccardi, C. (1994). Bifurcation analysis pf periodic SEIR and SIR epidemic models. *J Math Biol, 32*(2), 109-121. https://doi.org/10.1007/BF00163027.

Lekone, P. E., & Finkenstädt, B. F. (2006). Statistical Inference in a Stochastic Epidemic SEIR Model with Control Intervention: Ebola as a Case Study. *Biometrics, 62*(4), 1170-1177. https://doi.org/10.1111/j.1541-0420.2006.00609.x.

Letsa-Agbozo, J. K., Kumah, M. S., & Yao, D. J. I. (2016). Sir model of hepatitis B disease in the North Tongu district. *Int J Appl Res, 2*(11), 229-234.

Li, C. H., & Yousef, A. M. (2019). Bifurcation analysis of a network-based SIR epidemic model with saturated treatment function. *Chaos, 29*(3), 033129. https://doi.org/10.1063/1.5079631.

Li, J., Ma, Z., Brauer, F. (2007). Global analysis of discrete-time SI and SIS epidemic models. *Mathematical Biosciences and Engineering 4*(4), 699.

Li, T., Zhang, F., Liu, H., & Chen, Y. (2017). Threshold dynamics of an SIRS model with nonlinear incidence rate and transfer from infectious to susceptible. *J. Applied Mathematics Letters, 70*, 52-57. https://doi.org/10.1016/j.aml.2017.03.005.

Li, Y., & Cui, J. (2009). The effect of constant and pulse vaccination on SIS epidemic models incorporating media coverage. *Communications in Nonlinear Science and Numerical Simulation, 14*(5), 2353-2365. https://doi.org/10.1016/j.cnsns.2008.06.024.

Li, Y., Li, W.-T., & Lin, G. (2015). Damped oscillating traveling waves of a diffusive SIR epidemic model. *Applied Mathematics Letters, 46*, 89-93. https://doi.org/10.1016/j.aml.2015.02.011.

Lindquist, J., Ma, J., Van Den Driessche, P., & Willeboordse, F. H. (2011). Effective degree network disease models. *Journal of Mathematical Biology, 62*(2), 143-164. https://doi.org/10.1007/s00285-010-0331-2.

Liu, J., & Zhang, T. (2011). Epidemic spreading of an SEIRS model in scale-free networks. *Communications in Nonlinear Science and Numerical Simulation 16*(8), 3375-3384. https://doi.org/10.1016/j.cnsns.2010.11.019.

Liu, J. J. (2017). Bifurcation of a delayed SEIS epidemic model with a changing delitescence and nonlinear incidence rate. *Discrete Dynamics in Nature and Society, 2017*, Article Article ID 2340549. https://doi.org/10.1155/2017/2340549.

Liu, S., Poccia, S., Candan, K. S., Chowell, G., & Sapino, M. L. (2016). epiDMS: Data Management and Analytics for Decision-Making From Epidemic Spread Simulation Ensembles. *J Infect Dis, 214*(suppl_4), S427-S432. https://doi.org/10.1093/infdis/jiw305.

Liu, W.-M., Hethcote, H. W., & Levin, S. A. (1987). Dynamical behavior of epidemiological models with nonlinear incidence rates. *Journal of Mathematical Biology, 25*(4), 359-380.

Ma, Y., & Yu, X. (2020). Threshold dynamics of a stochastic SIVS model with saturated incidence and Lévy jumps. *Advances in Difference Equations. 2020*(1), 1-16. https://doi.org/10.1186/s13662-020-02723-9.

Maheshwari, P., & Albert, R. (2020). Network model and analysis of the spread of COVID-19 with social distancing. *Applied Network Science, 5*(1), 1-13.

Mateus, J. P., Rebelo, P., Rosa, S., Silva, C. M., & Torres, D. F. M. (2017). Optimal control of non-autonomous SEIRS models with vaccination and treatment. *American Institute of Mathematical Sciences, 11*(6), 1179-1199. https://doi.org/10.3934/dcdss.2018067.

Meng, X., Chen, L., & Cheng, H. (2007). Two profitless delays for the SEIRS epidemic disease model with nonlinear incidence and pulse vaccination. *Applied Mathematics and Computation, 186*(1), 516-529. https://doi.org/10.1016/j.amc.2006.07.124.

Meng, X., Wu, Z., & Zhang, T. (2013). The dynamics and therapeutic strategies of a SEIS epidemic model. *International Journal of Biomathematics, 6*(05), 1350029.

Meng, X., Zhao, S., Feng, T., & Zhang, T. (2016). Dynamics of a novel nonlinear stochastic SIS epidemic model with double epidemic hypothesis. *Mathematical Analysis and Applications, 433*(1), 227-242. https://doi.org/10.1016/j.jmaa.2015.07.056.

Menon, A., Rajendran, N. K., Chandrachud, A., & Setlur, G. (2020). Modelling and simulation of COVID-19 propagation in a large population with specific reference to India. *MedRxiv*. https://doi.org/10.1101/2020.04.30.20086306.

Mikolajczyk, R. T., & Kretzschmar, M. (2008). Collecting social contact data in the context of disease transmission: prospective and retrospective study designs. *Social Networks, 30*(2), 127-135.

Miller, J., & Ting, T. (2019). EoN (Epidemics on Networks): a fast, flexible Python package for simulation, analytic approximation, and analysis of epidemics on networks. *Journal of Open Source Software, 4*(44), 1731. https://doi.org/10.21105/joss.01731

Mohamadou, Y., Halidou, A., & Kapen, P. T. (2020). A review of mathematical modeling, artificial intelligence and datasets used in the study, prediction and management of COVID-19. *Applied Intelligence, 50*(11), 3913-3925. https://doi.org/10.1007/s10489-020-01770-9.

Mohammadi, H., Rezapour, S., & Jajarmi, A. (2021). On the fractional SIRD mathematical model and control for the transmission of COVID-19: The first and the second waves of the disease in Iran and Japan. *ISA Trans.* https://doi.org/10.1016/j.isatra.2021.04.012.

Momoh, A. A., Ibrahim, M. O., & Madu, B. A. (2011). Stability Analysis of an infectious disease free equilibrium of Hepatitis B model. *Research Journal of Applied Sciences, Engineering and Technology, 3*(9), 905-909.

Monteiro, N. Z., & Mazorche, S. R. (2021). Analysis and application of a fractional SIR model constructed with Mittag-Leffler distribution. *Proceedings of the XLII Ibero-Latin-American Congress on Computational Methods in Engineering.*

Muñoz-Fernández, G. A., Seoane, J. M., & Seoane-Sepúlveda, J. B. (2021). A SIR-type model describing the successive waves of COVID-19. *Chaos, Solitons & Fractals, 144*, 110682. https://doi.org/10.1016/j.chaos.2021.110682.

Naim, M., Lahmidi, F., & Namir, A. (2021). Threshold Dynamics of an $$\mathbf{SEIS}$$ Epidemic Model with Nonlinear Incidence Rates. *Differential Equations and Dynamical Systems.* https://doi.org/10.1007/s12591-021-00581-9.

Ngwa, G. A., & Teboh-Ewungkem, M. I. (2016). A mathematical model with quarantine states for the dynamics of ebola virus disease in human populations. *Computational and Mathematical Methods in Medicine,* 2016.

Olaniyi, S., Okosun, K. O., Adesanya, S. O., & Lebelo, R. S. (2020). Modelling malaria dynamics with partial immunity and protected travellers: optimal control and cost-effectiveness analysis. *Journal of Biological Dynamics, 14*(1), 90-115. https://doi.org/10.1080/17513758.2020.1722265.

Ostaszewski, M., Niarakis, A., Mazein, A., Kuperstein, I., Phair, R., Orta-Resendiz, A., Glaab, E. (2021). COVID19 Disease Map, a computational knowledge repository of virus–host interaction mechanisms. *Molecular Systems Biology, 17*(10), e10387.

Paladini, F., Renna, I., & Renna, L. (2011). A discrete sirs model with kicked loss of immunity and infection probability. *Journal of Physics: Conference Series.*

Pandey, G., Chaudhary, P., Gupta, R., & Pal, S. (2020). SEIR and Regression Model based COVID-19 outbreak predictions in India. *arXiv.* https://doi.org/10.48550/arXiv.2004.0095.

Park, D. J., Park, M. W., Lee, H., Kim, Y. J., Kim, Y., & Park, Y. H. (2021). Development of machine learning model for diagnostic disease prediction based on laboratory tests. *Sci Rep, 11*(1), 7567. https://doi.org/10.1038/s41598-021-87171-5.

Philemon, M. D., Ismail, Z., & Dare, J. (2019). A review of epidemic forecasting using artificial neural networks. *International Journal of Epidemiologic Research*, *6*(3), 132-143. https://doi.org/10.15171/ijer.2019.24.

Picault, S., Huang, Y.-L., Sicard, V., Arnoux, S., Beaunée, G., & Ezanno, P. (2019). EMULSION: Transparent and flexible multiscale stochastic models in human, animal and plant epidemiology. *PLOS Computational Biology*, *15*(9), e1007342. https://doi.org/10.1371/journal.pcbi.1007342.

Piret, J., & Boivin, G. (2021). Pandemics throughout history. *Frontiers in Microbiology*, 3594.

Prevention, C. F. D. C. A. (2018). Lesson 1: Introduction to Epidemiology, Section 11: Epidemic Disease Occurrence. *CDC*. Available online at: https://www.cdc.gov/csels/dsepd/ss1978/lesson1/section11.html.[Last accessed on 5th May, 2020].

Quirouette, C., Younis, N. P., Reddy, M. B., & Beauchemin, C. A. (2020). A mathematical model describing the localization and spread of influenza A virus infection within the human respiratory tract. *PLoS Computational Biology*, *16*(4), e1007705.

Qureshi, S., & Yusuf, A. (2019). Fractional derivatives applied to MSEIR problems: Comparative study with real world data. *The European Physical Journal Plus*, *134*(4). https://doi.org/10.1140/epjp/i2019-12661-7.

Rafiq, M., Ahmad, W., Abbas, M., & Baleanu, D. (2020). A reliable and competitive mathematical analysis of Ebola epidemic model. *Advances in Difference Equations*, *2020*(1), 1-24. https://doi.org/10.1186/s13662-020-02994-2.

Rao, F., Mandal, P. S., & Kang, Y. (2019). Complicated endemics of an SIRS model with a generalized incidence under preventive vaccination and treatment controls. *Applied Mathematical Modelling*, *67*, 38-61. https://doi.org/10.1016/j.apm.2018.10.016.

Ribassin-Majed, L., & Lounes, R. (2010). A SIS model for Human Papillomavirus transmission. *Mathematical Medicine and Biology: a Journal of the IMA*, *31*(2), 125-149.

Rifhat, R., Teng, Z., & Wang, C. (2021). Extinction and persistence of a stochastic SIRV epidemic model with nonlinear incidence rate. *Advances in Difference Equations*, *2021*(1). https://doi.org/10.1186/s13662-021-03347-3.

Sahu, G. P., & Dhar, J. (2012). Analysis of an SVEIS epidemic model with partial temporary immunity and saturation incidence rate. *Applied Mathematical Modelling*, *36*(3), 908-923.

Salathé, M., & Jones, J. H. (2010). Dynamics and control of diseases in networks with community structure. *PLoS Computational Biology*, *6*(4), e1000736.

Sanz, J., Xia, C.-Y., Meloni, S., & Moreno, Y. (2014). Dynamics of Interacting Diseases. *Physical Review X*, *4*(4). https://doi.org/10.1103/physrevx.4.041005.

Schurz, H., & Tosun, K. (2015). Stochastic asymptotic stability of SIR model with variable diffusion rates. *Journal of Dynamics and Differential Equations*, *27*(1), 69-82. https://doi.org/10.1007/s10884-014-9415-9.

Song, P., Lou, Y., & Xiao, Y. (2019). A spatial SEIRS reaction-diffusion model in heterogeneous environment. *Journal of Differential Equations*, *267*(9), 5084-5114.

Stolerman, L. M., Coombs, D., & Boatto, S. (2015). SIR-network model and its application to dengue fever. *SIAM Journal on Applied Mathematics*, *75*(6), 2581-2609. https://doi.org/http://www.jstor.org/stable/43895792.

Surya, L. (2018). How government can use AI and ML to identify spreading infectious diseases. *International Journal of Creative Research Thoughts, 6*(1), 2320-2882.

Syafruddin, S., & Noorani, M. S. M. (2012). SEIR model for transmission of dengue fever in Selangor Malaysia. *International Journal of Modern Physics Conference Series.*

Takeuchi, Y., Ma, W., & Beretta, E. (2000). Global asymptotic properties of a delay SIR epidemic model with finite incubation times. *Nonlinear Analysis, 42*(6), 931-947. https://doi.org/10.1016/S0362-546X(99)00138-8.

Taylor, R. A., Moore, C. L., Cheung, K.-H., & Brandt, C. (2018). Predicting urinary tract infections in the emergency department with machine learning. *PLOS ONE, 13*(3), e0194085. https://doi.org/10.1371/journal.pone.0194085.

Tolles, J., & Luong, T. (2020). Modeling Epidemics With Compartmental Models. *JAMA, 323*(24), 2515. https://doi.org/10.1001/jama.2020.8420.

Totaro, M. L. S. (*2008*). Analysis of an Age-Structured Mseir Model. *Del Seminario Matematico, 66*(2), 113.

Trawicki, M. (2017). Deterministic Seirs Epidemic Model for Modeling Vital Dynamics, Vaccinations, and Temporary Immunity. *Mathematics, 5*(1), 7. https://doi.org/10.3390/math5010007.

Tulu, T. W., Tian, B., & Wu, Z. (2017). Modeling the effect of quarantine and vaccination on Ebola disease. *Advances in Difference Equations, 2017*(1). https://doi.org/10.1186/s13662-017-1225-z.

Umar, M., Sabir, Z., Zahoor Raja, M. A., Gupta, M., Le, D.-N., Aly, A. A., & Guerrero-Sánchez, Y. (2021). Computational Intelligent Paradigms to Solve the Nonlinear SIR System for Spreading Infection and Treatment Using Levenberg–Marquardt Back-propagation. *Symmetry, 13*(4), 618. https://doi.org/10.3390/sym13040618.

Vardavas, R., Breban, R., & Blower, S. (2007). Can Influenza Epidemics Be Prevented by Voluntary Vaccination? *PLoS Computational Biology, 3*(5), e85. https://doi.org/10.1371/journal.pcbi.0030085.

Wan, H., & Cui, J. A. (2007). An SEIS epidemic model with transport-related infection. *J Theor Biol, 247*(3), 507-524. https://doi.org/10.1016/j.jtbi.2007.03.032.

Wang, P., & Jia, J. (2019). Stationary distribution of a stochastic SIRD epidemic model of Ebola with double saturated incidence rates and vaccination. *Advances in Difference Equations, 2019*(1). https://doi.org/10.1186/s13662-019-2352-5.

Wang, X. (2015). An SIRS Epidemic Model with Vital Dynamics and a Ratio-Dependent Saturation Incidence Rate. *Discrete Dynamics in Nature and Society, 2015*, 1-9. https://doi.org/10.1155/2015/720682.

White, L. A., Forester, J. D., & Craft, M. E. (2018). Dynamic, spatial models of parasite transmission in wildlife: Their structure, applications and remaining challenges. *Journal of Animal Ecology, 87*(3), 559-580. https://doi.org/10.1111/1365-2656.12761.

Widyaningsih, P., Candrawati, P., & Saputro, D. R. S. (2019). Maternal Antibody Susceptible Vaccinated Infected Recovered (MSVIR) Model for Tetanus Disease and Its Applications in Indonesia. *Journal of Physics: Conference Series.*

Willem, L., Verelst, F., Bilcke, J., Hens, N., & Beutels, P. (2017). Lessons from a decade of individual-based models for infectious disease transmission: a systematic review (2006-2015). *BMC Infectious Diseases, 17*(1), 1-16.

Wiratsudakul, A., Suparit, P., & Modchang, C. (2018). Dynamics of Zika virus outbreaks: an overview of mathematical modeling approaches. *PeerJ, 6*, e4526.

Xia, W., Kundu, S., & Maitra, S. (2018). Dynamics of a delayed SEIQ epidemic model. *Advances in Difference Equations, 2018*(1). https://doi.org/10.1186/s13662-018-1791-8.

Xu, R. (2012). Global dynamics of an SEIS epidemic model with saturation incidence and latent period. *Applied Mathematics and Computation, 218*(15), 7927-7938. https://doi.org/10.1016/j.amc.2012.01.076.

Yan, S., Zhang, Y., Ma, J., & Yuan, S. (2018). An edge-based SIR model for sexually transmitted diseases on the contact network. *J Theor Biol, 439*, 216-225. https://doi.org/10.1016/j.jtbi.2017.12.003.

Yang, B. (2016). Stochastic dynamics of an SEIS epidemic model. *Advances in Difference Equations, 2016*(1). https://doi.org/10.1186/s13662-016-0914-3.

Yang, Z., Zeng, Z., Wang, K., Wong, S.-S., Liang, W., Zanin, M., . . . He, J. (2020). Modified SEIR and AI prediction of the epidemics trend of COVID-19 in China under public health interventions. *Journal of Thoracic Disease, 12*(3), 165-174. https://doi.org/10.21037/jtd.2020.02.64.

Yokchoo, N., Patanarapeelert, N., & Patanarapeelert, K. (2019). The effect of group A streptococcal carrier on the epidemic model of acute rheumatic fever. *Theoretical Biology and Medical Modelling, 16*(1). https://doi.org/10.1186/s12976-019-0110-8.

Yu, Z., Arif, R., Fahmy, M. A., & Sohail, A. (2021). Self organizing maps for the parametric analysis of COVID-19 SEIRS delayed model. *Chaos Solitons Fractals, 150*, 111202. https://doi.org/10.1016/j.chaos.2021.111202.

Zewdie, A. D., & Gakkhar, S. (2020). A Mathematical Model for Nipah Virus Infection. *Journal of Applied Mathematics, 2020*, 1-10. https://doi.org/10.1155/2020/6050834.

Zhang, X., & Liu, X. (2009). Backward bifurcation and global dynamics of an SIS epidemic model with general incidence rate and treatment. *Abstract and Applied Analysis, 10*(2), 565-575. https://doi.org/10.1155/2012/647853.

Zhang, Z., & Si, F. (2014). Dynamics of a delayed SEIRS-V model on the transmission of worms in a wireless sensor network. *Advances in Difference Equations, 2014*(1), 295. https://doi.org/10.1186/1687-1847-2014-295.

Zhao, D., & Yuan, S. (2016). Persistence and stability of the disease-free equilibrium in a stochastic epidemic model with imperfect vaccine. *Advances in Difference Equations, 2016*(1). https://doi.org/10.1186/s13662-016-1010-4.

Zhao, D., Zhang, T., & Yuan, S. (2016). The threshold of a stochastic SIVS epidemic model with nonlinear saturated incidence. *Physica A: Statistical Mechanics and its Applications, 443*, 372-379. https://doi.org/10.1016/j.physa.2015.09.092.

Zhao, H., Jiang, J., Xu, R., & Ye, Y. (2014). SIRS Model of Passengers' Panic Propagation under Self-Organization Circumstance in the Subway Emergency. *Mathematical Problems in Engineering, 2014*, 1-12. https://doi.org/10.1155/2014/608315.

Zhou, X., & Cui, J. (2011). Analysis of stability and bifurcation for an SEIV epidemic model with vaccination and nonlinear incidence rate. *Nonlinear Dynamics, 63*(4), 639-653.

# Chapter 3

# Immunomodulation and Immunotherapy to Tackle Opportunistic Infections

## Sayed Muhammad Ata Ullah Bukhari[1], Liloma Shah[2], Sana Raza[2] and Muhsin Jamal[2,*]

[1]Department of Microbiology,
Quaid-I-Azam University, Islamabad, Pakistan
[2]Department of Microbiology,
Abdul Wali Khan University, Mardan, Pakistan

### Abstract

Opportunistic infections (OIs) are those that occur more frequently and severely in people with a weakened immune system. These infections are more severe as a result of the predisposing to other illnesses or their therapy. The causative agents of OIs are parasites, fungi, bacteria and viruses and such microbes take benefit of an opportunity that is ordinarily not available. These opportunities occur when the microbiome is altered leading to a weakened defense mechanism/ immune system or may be due to the usage of immune-suppressive medications. Several approaches have been developed to tackle OIs. There is a great need for innovative and novel approaches to be developed to overcome these challenges. Moreover, control and preventive measures should be taken to handle the emergence of resistance to drugs and drug toxicity. The suitable efficacy of drugs should be established to overcome such infections. As shown through current advances and accomplishments in the field of pharmaceuticals such as the development of monoclonal antibodies, immunotherapies have the potential to overcome these limitations. This chapter deals with various immunotherapies for tackling OIs. These

---

[*] Corresponding Author's Email: muhsinjamal@awkum.edu.pk, muhsinkhan08@gmail.com.

In: Interdisciplinary Approaches on Opportunistic Infections …
Editors: Jayapradha Ramakrishnan and Ganesh Babu Malli Mohan
ISBN: 978-1-68507-984-0
© 2022 Nova Science Publishers, Inc.

immunotherapies (adaptive and innate) include checkpoint inhibition, cytokine levels manipulation, mAb-based therapies, and T-cell-based therapies. To treat such infections a chief role is played by adaptive immunotherapy and immunotherapeutics would influence its extensive implementation.

**Keywords:** infections, immunotherapy, opportunistic, immunity

## 1. Introduction

Medical advancements have prolonged the lives of many people living with cancer, rheumatological disease, and solid organ and stem cell transplant recipients. However, many of the treatments weaken or alter the patient's immune system which makes the immune system suppressed and individually vulnerable to infections through opportunistic microbes (Gooley et al., 2010). Numerous drugs are developed against such opportunistic bacterial, fungal and viral infections (Corzo-Leon et al., 2015). Such a medications used against these infections are not only expensive and but also often associated with significant toxicity (Mahmoud et al., 2021). Additionally, resistance against antifungal, antibacterial, and antiviral agents is an emergent issue and can be linked with a higher probability of treatment failures (Campos et al., 2016). Therefore, it is important if particular anti-pathogen precise immunity is induced for controlling the infections. For example, T-cells play an important role against invasive viral infections (Tormo et al., 2011). Moreover, innate immunity also plays an important role in the control of infections caused by mould. Furthermore, for controlling bacterial infections, monoclonal antibodies (mAbs) are reconsidered (Motley et al., 2019). Apart from the above discussed immunotherapeutic approaches immunotherapies are also used to tackle opportunistic bacterial infections; like cytokine therapy, checkpoint inhibition and T-cell-based immunotherapies. The application of immunomodulatory substances also appears to be a striking strategy as an adjunct modality to manage numerous opportunistic infections caused by parasites (Luster et al., 2005).

Some of the fungal associated infections (i.e. histoplasmosis, penicilliosis, zygomycosis, cryptococcosis, aspergillosis, candidiasis), and other caused by *Sporothrix* spp., *Fusarium* spp. and *Scedoporium* spp. are much challenging to medicate. These invasive fungal diseases are the main reasons for substantial mortality and morbidity amongst immunocompromised individuals (Neofytos et al., 2009). Other disease-causing microbes and fungal species could be the reason for infections in general circumstances also called "virulence factors." These factors included: (i) capability of colonizing and/or invading the host cell; (ii) resistance to body temperature of the host; (iii) resistance to the immune system of the host and/or evading the immune system and (iv) secretion of the toxins and proteolytic enzyme (Pirofski and Casadevall 2015). In humans, higher mortality and morbidity rates are linked to fungal infections despite the accessibility of numerous antifungal medications (Brown et al., 2012). In such a situation, there is a dire need to develop novel effective and safe anti-fungal drugs to reduce the burden of fungal infections (Perfect 2016). At the very same time, there is an urgent need of immunotherapeutic approaches to restore immune system of the the host (Pflughoeft and Versalovic 2012). Apart from these fungal opportunistic infections, there are also some other OIs caused by bacteria, viruses and parasites.

Some of the important opportunistic infections such as progressive multifocal leukoencephalopathy (PML), respiratory infections, Kaposi sarcoma (a kind of cancer), toxoplasmosis infection and gastrointestinal tract (GIT) infections are caused *Bhuman Polyomavirus*-2, *Cytomegalovirus*, *Human Herpesvirus*-8, *Toxoplasma gondii*, and *Cryptosporidium* respectively. To handle the mentioned OIs, Immunomodulation and immunotherapy can play a vital role and offer a therapeutic modality to increase immune responses to limit this infection. In this chapter, we have discussed the principles of immunotherapy and immunomodulation against different opportunistic infections caused by fungi, bacteria, viruses and parasites infections (Table 1.1).

## 2. Immunotherapy

Immunotherapies help in the manipulation of the components of the immune system to target and eliminate microbes in order to protect the diseased individual. Immunotherapies are classified into the following 2 types based on their mode of action: (1) Active immunotherapies and (2) Passive immunotherapies. Active immunotherapies activate immunological memory components of the host by applying virulence factors that do the activation of effector's (humoral response or T-cells), while in passive immunotherapies ex-vivo made constituents are used (like derivatives of recombinant antibody and immune cells) that are administrated to patients (Papaioannou et al., 2016).

**Table 1.1.** Immunomodulation and immunotherapy to tackle opportunistic infections

| S/No | Agents | Microorganisms | Infections | Immunotherapy | References |
|---|---|---|---|---|---|
| 1 | Bacterial | *Clostridioides difficile* | Mild diarrhea to pseudomembranous colitis | Innate immune response phagocytosis, oxidative killing and cytokine mediated response Adaptive immune responses such as T- and B-lymphocyte mediated responses | Lessa et al., 2012, Abt MC et al., 2015 |
| | | *Legionella pneumophila* | Legionnaires' disease (severe form of pneumonia) | T and B cells are ultimately required for the clearance of the infection. Evidence for the role of T cells comes from the depletion of CD4 or CD8 T cells using monoclonal antibodies, | Brenner et al., 1979, Susa, et al., 1998. |
| | | *Mycobacterium avium complex* | Tuberculosis | rIL-12 | Silva, R.A., Pais, T.F. and Appelberg, R., 1998 |
| | | *Mycobacterium tuberculosis* | Tuberculosis | T cell response, IFN-γ-releasing $CD4^+$ T cells, cytotoxic $CD4^+$ T cell subsets (and $CD8^+$ T cells | Getahun et al., 2015; van de Berg et al., 2008. |
| | | *HSCT* | Severe nosocomial and community acquired infections at various body sites including the urinary tract, surgical or burn wounds, the cornea and the lower respiratory tract, cystic fibrosis | rhIL-7, anti-lipopolysaccharide (LPS) immunoglobulin M (IgM) monoclonal antibody | Do'ring et al. 2000; Driscoll et al., 2007; Que et al., 2014. |
| | | *Streptococcus pneumoniae* | Pneumococcal infections (Pneumonia) | IL-1 | Ludwig et al., 2012; Arend, 2002 |
| 2. | Viral | *Human Polyomavirus 2* | Fatal demyelinating disease | T-cell responses | Elphick et al., 2004. Davies, Sarah L; Muranski, Pawel (2017). |
| | | *Human herpesvirus 8* | Kaposi's sarcoma. 2 | cytotoxic T lymphocytes (CTL) | Martin et al. (1998); Micheletti et al., 2002. |

| S/No | Agents | Microorganisms | Infections | Immunotherapy | References |
|---|---|---|---|---|---|
| 3. | Fungal | *Aspergillus conidia* | Invasive pulmonary aspergillosis | Granulocytes, antigen-specific T cells as well as the administration of recombinant cytokines and growth factors (e.g., interferon-$\gamma$ (IFN-$\gamma$), granulocyte- and granulocyte-macrophage colony stimulating factor (G-CSF, GM-CSF), TNF-$\alpha$, IL-15) | Latgé, J.P., 1999; Medici NP, Del Poeta M 2015 |
| 4. | Parasitic | *Cryptosporidium parvum* | Cryptosporidiosis (diarrhea) | Innate (toll-like receptors TLRs) and adaptive immunity FN-$\gamma$ or IL-4 and IL-5 CD4+ T cells | Putignani L, Menichella D (2010); Chen XM, O'Hara SP, Nelson JB et al. (2005); Riggs MW (2002) Flanigan T, Whalen C, Turner J (1992) |
| | | *Toxoplasma gondii* | Toxoplasmosis | Toll-like receptors (TLRs) | Chen K et al., 2007). |

Vaccines are the oldest and most successful form of immunotherapy (Naran et al., 2018) which normally protects against microbes through the following ways i.e., (i) "immunological memory via administrating immunogens for inducing clonal proliferation of antigen-specific lymphocytes, permitting the immune system of the host to respond much quickly and efficiently (Janeway et al., 2001) and (ii) "conferring passive protection, post-infection, through delivering neutralizing agents like antibodies binding (Naran et al., 2018). Communicable diseases like polio and smallpox are completely eradicated using immunization. In the previous three decades, advancements in science resulted in the development of newer vaccine platforms applying nucleic acid-based vaccines and recombinant antibodies (Rappuoli et al., 2014). For therapeutic purposes, the mAbs are permitted since 1986 and presently they are extensively used in immunotherapies. Monoclonal antibodies perform their roles in different ways such as i.e., (i) they bind to receptors that are present on the surface of the cell and induce a cascade of signals, and cause cell death; (ii) interfering with the ligand-receptor associations required for viability or continued growth of cell; (iii) inducing antibody-dependent cellular cytotoxicity, that comprises the antibody Fc region serving to recruit cell-mediated immunity constituents [like macrophages, monocytes and natural killer (NK) cells] and (iv) through complement-dependent cytotoxicity which arises from complement cascade activation afterward attaching to the targeted structure. Moreover, the targeting domain of monoclonal antibody which is bonded to toxic payload is used by antibody conjugates to target antigens that are associated with the disease. By binding to the target, internalization occurs, and the payload is released which triggered the death of the cell (Naran et al., 2018).

At present-specific antibodies containing 2 binding domains (one specific for effector cell while the other for an antigen) has also been developed. In this way, multiple ligands/receptors are interfered with by such antibodies and molecules involved within inflammatory processes or cell proliferation (Suurs et al., 2019). Currently, checkpoint blockade therapy is the most prominent immunotherapy. In this therapy, the immune system of the host is prevented to attack healthier cells extensively using immune checkpoints. Notable checkpoint-blockade monoclonal antibodies attack T-cell immunoglobulin, mucin domain-containing protein-3 (TIM3), programmed cell death protein-1 (PD1), cytotoxic T-lymphocyte-associated protein-4 (CTLA-4) and programmed cell death 1 ligand 1 (PD-L1) that avoid inhibition of T-cells resulting in its activation. In 2011, US Food and Drug Administration (FDA) approved several inhibitors of checkpoints for treating different cancers.

Positive results were obtained when they were used in combination with other therapies against malaria, tuberculosis (TB), and human immunodeficiency virus (HIV).

Apart from the inhibitors, cytokines were also approved for therapeutic purposes in 1986 (Riley et al., 2019). These are soluble proteins that facilitate intercellular communications for numerous bio-logical mechanisms comprising proliferation of the cell, wound healing, inflammation, angiogenesis, and immunity. Signaling is mediated by cytokines which are essential both for controlling and spread of disease. Another immunotherapeutic approach is chimeric antigen receptor (CAR-T) cell immunotherapy. It enhances the function of T-cells using chimeric antigen receptor T-cells (CAR-T) (Naran et al., 2018).

## 3. Immunotherapy and Immunomodulation to Tackle Different Opportunistic Infections

To tackle OIs different immunotherapies and immunomodulation are used. Following are the immunomodulation and immunotherapies for tackling different opportunistic infections caused by fungi, viruses, bacteria, and parasites.

### 3.1. Immunotherapy to Tackle Fungal Opportunistic Infections

OIs are still a great health issue. Annually 1.6 million deaths are caused by opportunistic fungal infections in immunocompromised individuals (Almeida et al., 2019). Due to no rapid and reliable diagnostic techniques and limited availability of antifungals for treating such opportunistic fungal infections (McCarthy et al., 2017). Individuals with extended neutropenia, solid organ transplant (SOT), allogeneic hematopoietic stem cell transplant (HSCT), acquired or inherited immunodeficiencies like AIDS patients or those who are using corticosteroids, so are at high risk to develop severe invasive fungal infections (IFIs) (White et al., 2017). Though *Aspergillus conidia* are present abundantly and each individual inhale about hundreds of them every day, due to the occurrence of phagocytic cells within the lungs and mucociliary clearance the immunocompetent persons are protected.

Consequently, within immune-compromised hosts invasive fungal infections are highly observed. Mostly fungi belonging *Aspergillus*, *Candida*, *Pneumocystis* or *Cryptococcus* genera are responsible for causing invasive fungal infections (Lauruschkat et al., 2018). Currently, three classes of antifungal drugs such as echinocandins (caspofungin), polyenes (amphotericin B, AmB), and azoles (fluconazole) are so for accessible for clinical application (Mor et al., 2015). The occurrence of mycoses is increasing due to the raising usage of immunomodulatory medications for treating cancer, autoimmune diseases, and recipients of transplants (Lauruschkat et al., 2018). Moreover, reports on the worldwide occurrence of resistance to antifungals particularly within *Aspergillus* spp. and *Candida* spp. highlighted the restricted treatment choices and the crucial necessity for innovative approaches to improve individuals who have invasive fungal infections (Hendrickson et al., 2019).

Since adaptive and innate responses of the immune system perform an important part in providing defense against infection caused by fungi, so, therefore, more investigators get curious about establishing adjunctive or novel approaches which enhance humoral and cellular functions within the host for improving the outcome of patients (Lauruschkat et al., 2018). Neutrophils and alveolar macrophages are phagocytic cells that perform an important role in removing the invading microbes within the lungs (Brown 2011). Numerous intra- and extracellular pattern recognition receptors (PRRs) are expressed immune cells of the innate system. Such PRRs not only help in the recognition of antigens associated with fungi but also regulate regulatory and proinflammatory responses (Wuthrich et al., 2012). Such properties enable the immune cells of the innate system as hopeful therapeutic targets. Some of the strategies for strengthening and modulating the immune system of the host include i.e., antibodies (abs), granulocyte and granulocyte-macrophage colony-stimulating factors (G-CSF, GM-CSF), growth factors and recombinant cytokines administration. Moreover, treatment of immunecompromised individuals could be done by cell therapy strategies that encompass transfusion of adaptive and innate immune cells for enhancing antifungal immunity.

### *3.1.1. Recombinant Cytokines and Immune Activating Compounds as Immune-Therapeutic Approach in Fungal Diseases*

Recombinant cytokines are another host-directed remedy that strengthens immunity and fights infections caused by fungi. Furthermore, increased sensitivity to fungal infections frequently arises from defects in the immune system such as acquired or primary immunodeficiencies (Wuthrich et al.,

2012). Interferon-γ (IFNγ) and recombinant colony-stimulating factors (CSFs) are used for reinforcing defense mechanisms against fungi.

### *3.1.2. Colony-Stimulating Factors*

It is a predisposing factor for fungal OIs when defects occur in neutrophils and to counter such defects, recombinant CSFs are applied as an adjunct remedy to stimulate and raise neutrophils to boost immune responses of the host to fungal microbes. For augmenting neutrophils, the recombinant kinds of G-CSF and GM-CSF are mainly applied but likewise, activation and proliferation of other myeloid cell-like circulating monocytes, dendritic cells (DCs), macrophages, eosinophils or platelets are FDA approved (Scriven et al., 2017). Within animal investigations, when GM-CSF was used combinedly with recombinant IFNγ or when used separately, it increased the fungicidal action of innate phagocytic cells (dendritic cells, macrophages, neutrophils) (Roilides et al., 1996).

Besides the fungicidal impacts observed within murine models, rapid neutrophils renewal, lessening of the burden of fungi within the lung of the immunosuppressed mouse, or macrophage suppression inhibition via corticosteroids dexamethasone or cortisone acetate were verified afterward G-CSF and GM-CSF were administered (Quezada et al., 2008). When G-CSF treatment was carried out jointly with caspofungin/amphotericin B intralipid or caspofungin in a murine model infected with *A. fumigatus*, satisfactory results were observed (Sionov et al., 2005).

FDA has approved both CSFs and G-CSFs not only for restoring the count of neutrophils but also for reducing neutropenia in patients with stem cell transplantation (Wright et al., 2017). Additionally, in animal experiments, G-CSF or GM-CSF appeared inspiring. Similarly, investigations concerning curing invasive fungal infections in human beings appeared satisfactory too. Safdar et al. examined the rhGM-CSF usage within immunosuppressive individuals with invasive fungal infections in which the administered usage of GM-CSF was well-tolerated and found safe. (Safdar et al., 2013). Moreover, the patients on antineoplastic therapy displayed the best outcomes after GM-CSF treatment (Wan et al., 2015). Furthermore, the results were more compromised when antifungal micafungin was co-administered with GM-CSF in a patient who was infected by *Scedosporium apiospermum*, (Chen et al., 2017).

### 3.1.3. IFNγ

IFNγ has shown the antifungal property by promoting naive $CD_{4+}$ T cells polarization to Th1 cells (helper cell type). Besides the polarization of Th1, IFNγ applied a positive impact on the fungicidal and fungistatic actions of neutrophils. Similarly, in-vitro production of $O_2$ was also mediated by it from PMNs afterward infection caused by *Pneumocystis carinii* (Buddingh et al., 2015). Moreover, pro-inflammatory cytokines production was raised within patients who suffered from invasive fungal infections. Further, it raised the production of TIL-22 and IL-1β by co-treatment with IFNγ and antifungals (Delsing et al., 2014).

Above mentioned factors show that they have a defensive role in increasing the anti-fungal activities. For example, Th22, Th17, and Th1 activation, bring improvement in functions of barrier and are also involved in the mobilization of neutrophils. Further study on patients who had undergone renal transplantation and suffered from invasive fungal infections showed effective treatment with IFNγ and AmB (Armstrong et al., 2010). Likewise, in recipients of allogeneic stem cell transplantation, the recombinant IFNγ has proven to be safe (Safdar et al., 2005). Patients who were not responding to anti-fungal medications and had cerebral cryptococcosis, in such patients IFNγ was utilized as rescue therapy. Complete clearance of *Cryptococci* was observed when IFNγ was co-administered with antifungals (Jarvis et al., 2012) and such study has shown that IFNγ has protective roles against fungal infections.

### 3.1.4. TNF-α

TNF-α is the utmost effective innate cytokine against *Aspergillus* (Jarvis et al., 2012). In a study, a mouse with invasive fungal infection was treated with TNF-α and its mortality rate was decreased (Nagai et al., 1995). Apart from the above-mentioned study, another investigation on TNF-α has shown its protective role when treatment was done in neutropenic and non-neutropenic mice. TNF-α raised the level of PMNs resulting in lungs infiltration and reduced the rate of mortality (Mehrad et al., 1999).

### 3.1.5. Other Cytokines

Several other cytokines also participate in the immune process throughout fungal infections, and these might be used in the future as immunotherapeutic agents. At multiple levels, IL-7 performs its role in improving the immunity of the host and it is an effective immunotherapeutic agent. When the mice infected with *C. albicans* were treated intravenously with IL-7 resulted in weakening of infection and improvement in the survival rate (Unsinger et al., 2012).Similarly, in *Paracoccidioides brasiliensis* and *Cryptococcus neoformans*, IL-18 showed a protective role (Ketelut et al., 2015).

### 3.1.6. Dendritic Cell Therapy

A bridge (dendritic cells) (DCS) is found between the adaptive and innate immune system. DCs sensed fungal microbes using PRRs and phagocytized the fungal particles. After processing these fungal particles, chemokines and cytokines are secreted into the surrounding followed by antigen presentation to cells for inducing an adaptive response of the immune system (Ramirez 2012). Such notable practical elasticity of DCs has been discovered for developing fungal vaccines (Roy and Klein 2012). Similarly, studies have shown induction of the adoptive immunity to *Aspergillus* using dendritic cells pulsed with alive conidia or transfected with conidial-RNA (Bozza et al., 2003). DCs primed with "CpGoligodeoxynucleotides" and pulsed with "Aspf16 antigens" (Bozza et al., 2002) activate protective and specific Th1 responses within murine models of hematopoietic stem cell transplantation (HSCT). Moreover, DCs transduction was done with a vector of adenovirus and it encoded the cDNA of IL-12 and pulsed with heat-inactivated *A. fumigatus* inducing a defensive response (higher rate of survival and reduced burdens of fungi) against invasive pulmonary aspergillosis model (Shao et al., 2005). Furthermore, defense against candidiasis within mice was observed with dendritic cells pulsed with proteins of cell wall expressed during infection, predominantly those obtained from fructose bisphosphate aldolase, that persuaded a vigorous defensive response against *C. albicans* (Xin et al., 2008).

### 3.1.7. Granulocyte Transfusion (GTX)

In blood stream, a particular type of cell is found called polymorphonuclear leukocytes. Using phagocytosis, such cells attack directly on microbes, and soluble anti-microbial substances are released which play an important role in providing defense against opportunistic fungal and bacterial infections (West et al., 2017). Patients suffering from extended neutropenia and severe infections are normally resistant to traditional treatment and can only be treated with granulocyte transfusion which results in improved granulocyte repopulation (Ang and Linn 2011). Pedersen et al. (1979) stated that pneumonia caused by *Pneumocystis carinii was* successfully when treated when granulocyte transfusion was used jointly with trimethoprim-sulfamethoxazole.

### 3.1.8. Adoptive T Cell Transfer

An artificial rise of fungal-specific T cells afterward the allogeneic hematopoietic stem cell transplantation may help in the clearance of *Aspergillus* in immune-compromised persons as they are much more vulnerable to fungal infections. In a study (in-vitro) when clones of *Aspergillus*-specific T cells were transferred to patients who had undergone allo-SCT and possessed uncontrolled invasive fungal infections resulted in hopeful outcomes in such patients (Perruccio et al., 2005).

In such immunotherapy the conservative T cells and Treg were co-infused. It not only provided immunity against fungal infections but also fatal graft-versus-host illness was prevented. One more option is the use of "gamma/delta (γδ) T cells" that do recognition of primarily diverse ligands from the shorter peptides which are seen via "alpha/beta (α/β) T cells" within the context of MHC class II or class I molecules. Anti-*Aspergillus* action is also shown by such cells (Srivastava et al., 2015). Numerous cytokines are secreted by γδ T cells and also such cells exert a cytotoxic effect. In addition to it, these cells are also involved in linking adaptive and innate immunity by complement systems or DCs (Kunzmann et al., 2009). Therefore, γδ T-cells adoptive transfer might be a hopeful candidate for treating invasive fungal infections.

### 3.1.9. Natural Killer Cell Therapy

Natural killer (NK) cells of humans were revealed to be operative against a broader range of fungal species like *Rhizopus oryzae* (Schmidt et al., 2013), *C. albicans* (Voigt et al., 2014) and *Aspergillus fumigatus* (Schneider et al., 2016). NK cells show their anti-fungal potential by direct mediators such as granzyme and perforin (Schmidt et al., 2011). Higher levels of NK cells are associated with better control of invasive infections in those patients who have undergone allo-SCT (Stuehler et al., 2015). Meanwhile, NK cell remedy is currently in its trial phase for cancer. Nonetheless, no clinical trial exists so far applying natural killer cells for treatment. However, there exists a higher capability of NK cell remedy as an immunotherapeutic choice for invasive fungal infection.

### 3.1.10. Antibody-Based Therapy

Immunoglobulins (antibodies) are proteins of heterodimeric nature consisting of two light and two heavy chains. These proteins provide defense against numerous diseases and are linked with particularly humoral immunity. Immunoglobulins play a protective role during fungal infections that could be achieved through direct and indirect processes (Casadevall and Pirofski 2012). The curiosity about the probable advantage of antibody-based remedies for fungal infections begins with Dromer et al. (Dromer et al., 19870). It was described that when monoclonal IgG1 anti-*Cryptococcus* antibody was administered intraperitoneally and might be utilized as passive sero-remedy. Furthermore, mAb M5E312 (a type of monoclonal antibody) effectively hindered the establishment of *P. carinii* infection within the experimental murine (Gigliotti and Hughes 1988). In addition, two monoclonal antibodies (18B7&Efungumab) have been used against fungi and are assessed in clinical trials.

### *3.1.11. Novel Approaches*

Small molecular therapeutics (SMTs) which help in the regulation, blocking or inhibition of the host signaling pathways have been extensively used in patients suffering from cancer. Immunosuppressive drugs and SMTs are received by such patients for down-regulating the immunity of hosts who are at higher risk of invasive fungal infections. The SMTs are also extensively used treatment of patients with autoimmune disorders (i.e., rheumatoid arthritis and systemic lupus erythematosus), who are also at increased risk of fungal infections (Mellinghoff et al., 2019). Moreover, the usage of non-TK inhibitors, tyrosine-protein kinase (TK) inhibitors, autophagy regulators and mammalian target of rapamycin (mTOR) was linked with reduced anti-fungal immunity. Beneficial effects are shown by checkpoint inhibitors in early infection of *Aspergillus* (D'Alessio et al., 2009).

PD-1/PD-L1 complex acts as checkpoint of the immune system via reducing immune responses and promoting tolerance (Okazaki and Wang 2005). In early infection caused by *A. fumigatus*, PD-L1 has shown persuade tolerance within dendritic cells, that outcome in up-regulating CTLA-4 activity and autoinflammatory cytokines secretion (Stephen et al., 2017). Hence in future, checkpoint-inhibitors might be proven as hopeful immunotherapeutic agent, not merely to cure autoinflammatory or malignant illnesses but also a potential candidate for fungal infections.

### 3.2. Immunotherapy to Tackle Bacterial Opportunistic Infections

*Clostridioides difficile, Legionella pneumophila, Mycobacterium avium complex, Mycobacterium tuberculosis, Pseudomonas aeruginosa, Staphylococcus aureus, Streptococcus pneumoniae* are a group of bacterial species which are accountable for OIs. To tackle OIs caused by these bacteria immunotherapeutic and Immunomodulatory approaches are used.

### 3.2.1. Monoclonal Antibody Therapy

Monoclonal antibodies have been used for the treatment of opportunistic infections caused by bacteria (Motley et al., 2019). During tuberculosis (TB), a significant role is played by the antibodies in immunomodulation and this is proved via the profiles of antibodies during latent TB infection that displayed improved "Fc-mediated immune effector" functions which carried out intracellular destruction of microbes via the macrophages. This function of antibodies highlighted their defensive role (Lu et al., 2016). Numerous monoclonal antibodies for *S. aureus* and *P. aeruginosa* have been engineered are in clinical trials. A bi-specific IgG1 antibody "MEDI3902 (AstraZeneca PLC)" is in the developmental phase for preventing pneumonia in higher-risk individuals. It targets the Psl exopolysaccharide (which is essential for adherence to tissues and colonization) and "PcrV protein" (which is vital for host cell cytotoxicity) (Ali et al., 2019). During a study when the patients with methicillin-resistant *S. aureus* (MRSA) were given the AR-301 (Aridis Pharmaceuticals), it resulted in providing defense against host cell damage mediated by alpha-toxin. AR-301 was a monoclonal antibody with alpha-toxin (virulence factor) neutralizing ability. Efficient immuno-prophylaxis was offered by a long-operative and novel mAb (MEDI4893) against *S. aureus* (AstraZeneca PLC)." It is in phase-2 clinical trials.

### 3.2.2. Cellular Therapies

Numerous studies have been performed to apply cellular therapies for treating bacterial infections. Transfer of macrophages could likewise be done adoptively for fighting infections caused by bacteria. In a study monocyte-derived macrophages (MDMs) were administered to murine models of *P. aeruginosa*, MRSA and *K. pneumoniae*. The load of bacterial species was reduced effectively when the intraperitoneal injection was used (Tacke et al., 2019). Recently, a system has been established for generating macrophages from human "induced pluripotent stem cells (iPSCs)" and stirred bioreactors have been applied in this process. When such cells were given intranasally, they effectively rescued the mice from an acute lung infection caused by *P. aeruginosa* (Ackermann et al., 2018).

### 3.2.3. T-Cell-Based Immunotherapies

It is very important to develop an effective treatment for TB (without or with co-infection of HIV.T-cells [HLA-E-restricted T-cells, γδ T-cells, mucosal-associated invariant T-cells (MAIT), and natural killer T-cells (NKT)] – a diverse T- lymphocytes class which are not confined to recognition of antigen using MHC – can be used as candidates within the establishment of immunotherapies which are T-cell based against the control of TB (La et al., 2020). Numerous lipids which are related to the cell of mycobacterium are recognized by the invariant natural killer T-cells (iNKT) and diverse kinds of cytokines (IL-21, IL-17A, IL-4, and IFN-γ) are produced by it which provoke immune responses against TB (Langan et al., 2020). In TB patients the efficiency of invariant natural killer T-cells is studied in phase- I and II clinical trials (NCT03551795).

### 3.2.4. Targeting Immune Checkpoints in Bacterial Infection

Programmed cell death protein 1 (PD-1), cells of the immune system like innate lymphoid cells (ILCs), innate lymphocytes (NK cells), and adaptive lymphocytes (B and T cells) perform an important part in eradicating and controlling infections. Such immune cells kill the infected cells and also inflammatory factors are secreted by it which reboots or increases myeloid bactericidal responses. Though, during infection, numerous stimuli are generated which up-regulate the molecules of the immune regulatory checkpoint.

When taking into consideration the evolutionary significance of such processes, like the main "T cell checkpoint inhibitory pathway PD-1/PD-L1," they are considered to avoid immune response over activation which could reason for harmful impacts such as damage to tissue and intensified inflammation. For instance, during infection of MTB, the PD-1 is upregulated on T-cells which seems important for avoiding immune-facilitated pathology. Though numerous disease-causing microorganisms, comprising pathogenic bacterial species, could take benefit of pathways that are immune-regulatory, and by this means the immune system is subverted by them (Wykes and Lewin 2018).

When such pathways are blocked it might be a feasible option to restore the function of immune cells for fighting infection. *Burkholderia* is bacteria that cause chronic infections and showed intrinsic resistance to numerous drugs. Due to such reasons, infections caused by this bacterium are difficult to be treated which can lead to death.PD-1 was upregulated on adaptive and innate immune cells by numerous smaller-colony variants of *B. pseudomallei* in the diseased murine models (See et al., 2017). Additionally, in the in-vitro infection model, the PD-L1 (ligand for PD-1) was upregulated on neutrophils of humans by *B. pseudomallei*. Production of IFN-γ and proliferation of T-cells were inhibited by it and also PD-1 was inhibited (Buddhisa et al., 2015). Such "PD-1/ PD-L1" process probably supports the persistence of infection. When such a pathway is blocked can help in the clearance of bacteria in such challenging infections.

Similarly, on T-cells, the PD-1 was up-regulated during *H. pylori* infection (Wu et al., 2011). In an in-vitro model of *H. pylori* infection, the PD-L1 was blocked so it reasoned for enhanced "CD4+ T cell-mediated" IL-2 production, which is a chief survival and proliferation factor for innate and adaptive lymphocytes (Das et al., 2006). Such PD-1/PD-L1 upregulation is proposed to be a key factor contributing to immune evasion via pre-malignant lesions throughout the establishment of gastric cancer (induced by *H. pylori*) (Shen et al., 2019). Both in infectious diseases and in cancer, the blockade and upregulation of PD-1 is the furthermost considered checkpoint. Though, data are progressively evolving which revealed that further checkpoints of the immune system such as Tim-3 i.e., "T cell immunoglobulin and mucin domain-containing protein 3," might have substantial support for illness (Triantafyllou et al., 2021).

### *3.2.5. T-Cell Immunoglobulin and Mucin Domain-Containing Protein 3 (Tim-3)*

During TB infection anti-PD1 therapies are carried out and the Tim-3 blockade seems to be much more hopeful. Just like PD-1, "Tim-3" is also a receptor of immune checkpoint and it is expressed on natural killer cells and T-cells. When it binds to its ligand i.e., galectin-9, it provides an inhibitory signal (Das et al., 2017). Both on murine and human T-cells the expression of Tim-3 is upregulated during infection through MTB (Jayaraman et al., 2016). In human CD8+ T cells, expression of Tim-3 was linked with lower production of IFN-and degranulation, the restoration could be done when anti-Tim-3 blocking antibodies were added (Das et al., 2017). The Tim-3 was upregulated by CD8+ T cells and CD4+ cells in a murine model of TB. Anti-Tim-3 blocking antibodies and Tim-3 knockout mice were applied for signifying that Tim-3 was a probable target that contributes for the persistence to bacteria (Jayaraman et al., 2016).

The above-mentioned study did not show the probable contribution of Tim-3 signaling within NK cells. The NK cells from an affected person with active or latent infection of TB have enhanced expression of Tim-3, which is adversely associated with the production of IFN-γ in reply to IL-12 (a characteristic IFN-γ trigger) (Wang et al., 2015). So far, the contribution of upregulation of Tim-3 on NK cells within a murine model of TB is not evaluated, and for additional studies, it is leftovers as a hopeful avenue. Alternatively, on macrophages, the expression of Tim-3 helps *Listeria monocytogenes* in evading the immune system. It inhibits the macrophage major histocompatibility complex (MHC-I) expression and then attenuates the production of CD8+ T cell responses (Wang et al., 2020). The blockade of Tim-3 might be an emergent treatment option against chronic infections for boosting immunity.

### *3.2.6. Cytokine Therapy*

Cytokine therapies have contributing roles in important biological mechanisms and numerous cytokines manipulation is done so far to alter the states of disease (Naran et al., 2018). It is shown by an in-vivo preclinical study that how innovative "albumin-fused granulocyte-macrophage colony-stimulating factor (GM-CSF)" enlarged the populations of dendritic cells which are accountable for producing effective immune responses against *M. tuberculosis* (Chuang et al., 2020). Additionally, in MDR TB-affected persons the recombinant human interleukin-2 (rhIL-2) is in clinical assessment and it is a type of adjunctive immunotherapy. It aims to shorten the course of treatment and improve the efficiency of treatment.

### *3.2.7. Emerging Technologies against Bacterial Pathogens*

The development of numerous innovative therapies is under consideration against bacterial infections. Conjugates of "antibody-antibiotic" enable the antibiotics targeted delivery. "DSTA4637S (Genentech), is an anti-*S. aureus* antibody antibiotic conjugates." It consists of a band used specifically against the cell wall teichoic acid of *S. aureus*. It is conjugated with antibiotics and a favorable pharmacokinetic profile and safety are shown by it within phase-1 clinical trials (Peck et al., 2019). Additionally, immunobiotics (synthetic), comprising of polymyxin-B (a drug that binds to the Gram-negative bacterial surface) and linked/conjugated with antibody-recruiting antigenic epitopes for inducing specific immune responses are under study (Feigman et al., 2018). Such investigations are promising for treating bacterial infections in the future.

## 3.3. Immunotherapy to Tackle Parasitic Opportunistic Infections

The following immunotherapies are used for tackling opportunistic infections caused by parasites.

### 3.3.1. Cytokines as Immunomodulatory Agents

Numerous cytokines activate the other cytokines production and are involved in antagonistic or synergistic networks (Masihi 2000). Recent advancements in cloning and identification by applying recombinant DNA technologies and monoclonal antibodies led to the accessibility of sufficient amounts of cytokines showing immunomodulatory activity. During parasitic infections, improper immunity is frequently linked with lowered IFN-γ, and also during such infections, the Th1 cytokine response is down-regulated. During infection caused by intracellular microbes, the IL-10 (i.e., Interleukin-10) is considered a fundamental mediator of the IFN-γ response which is depressed during these infections (Gong et al., 1996).

To organize suitable cytokine responses, the "T-helper lymphoid cells" are vital. IL-2, TNF-α and IFN-γ are produced by Th1 cells and these are needed for effectively producing the cell-mediated immune responses against intracellular pathogens. IL-5 and IL-4 are produced by Th2 cells which boost humoral immunity against those antigens which are T-dependent, and these cells are needed for producing immunity against infections caused by helminth. During the last decade, numerous studies have been conducted on cytokines. Several studies have been done to investigate the impacts of novel cloned cytokines within infectious illness mechanisms in the past decades (Hubbell et al., 2009).

### 3.3.2. Check Point Blockade

When monoclonal antibodies (mAbs) were used for blocking the interaction of PD1/PD-L1, they effectively treated leishmaniasis and malaria in mice. When mAbs were applied against the PD-1 receptor, they targeted PD-L1 and CD4+ lymphocytes within dendritic cells in both illnesses. These investigations highlighted the treatment capabilities of these antibodies (da Fonseca-Martins et al., 2019). On the other side, the protective role was shown by PD-L2 in malarial infection via inhibiting the interaction of PD1/PD-L1 and Th1 immunity (Wykes et al., 2018).

### 3.3.3. Interleukins

NK cells and T-cells are stimulated directly by IL-12 which produces IFN-γ. Macrophages are activated by IFN-γ and it is the reason for the resolution of disease. Malarial infection was effectively treated by recombinant IL-12. During the initial 5-6 days of infection, when treatment was carried out, so it lowered the parasitemia peak, and the onset of parasitemia was delayed by it. Lethal infection was prevented within the mice sensitive to *P. chabaudi* (Muniz- 2007). Malarial anemia was also effectively corrected by IL-12 (Stevenson et al., 2001). It is shown by a study that within the co-culture system of NK cell/ macrophage, IL- 18 and IL-12 enabled the generation of higher concentrations of TNF and IFN-γ for successively inducing macrophage anti-leishmanial actions (Prajeeth et al., 2011). Apart from this, IL-10 (i.e., Interleukin-10) is a cytokine that is immunomodulatory in action. Numerous cells are responsible for its production comprising thymocytes, macrophages, activated Th2 cells, monocytes, keratinocytes, and B cells.

An important role is played by IL-10 in establishing and maintaining immune response via augmenting immune responses which are Th2-dependent and suppressing Th1- dependent cell-mediated immunity (Mosmann and Moore 1991). IL-10 via indirect interactions prevents antigen-specific T-cell proliferation, stimulation, and production of cytokines and indirectly it reduces monocytes Ag presenting capability. *L. donovani* persuades endogenic production of murine IL-10, which sequentially enables the existence of protozoan intracellularly (Bhattacharyya et al., 2001). With neutralizing anti-IL-10 mAbs, when the infected macrophages were pre-incubated, it blocked both nitric oxide inhibition and release of TNF-α via the infected macrophages.

### 3.3.4. Antibody Conjugates

The utmost straight evidence of infectious illness profiting from immunotherapy of cancer could be illustrated by applying the instance of MacGregor and coworkers who verified in- vitro killing and receptor-dependent internalization of *Trypanosoma brucei* utilizing "human haptoglobin hemoglobin receptor (HpHbR) mAbs" conjugated to a "pyrrolobenzodiazepine toxin" (MacGregor et al., 2019).

### 3.3.5. Interferons

During chronic and acute stages of infection, host resistance is mediated by IFN-γ. It also protects against numerous intracellular microbes. Principally IFN-γ is a Th1-effector cytokine that directly shows the inhibitory impact on

Th-2 cytokines (Leonardo et al., 2005). By macrophages and dendritic cells, it induces the production of IL-12 (Szabo et al., 2000). Several experimental investigations have verified the significant role of IFN-γ in protecting against numerous infections. Applicable experimental information and emergent clinical outcomes recommended that IFN-γ, a "T-cell-derived lymphokine" has a broader macrophage activating impact and it also potentially treats non-viral infections. IFN-γ is a cytokine that enhances host defense, and its clinical potential is still unexplored. When IFN-γ is used in combination with traditional anti-monial medication, it effectively treats not only visceral leishmaniasis but also other kinds of cutaneous leishmaniasis (Murray et al., 1994).

In a study, IFN-γ was used in T-cell-deficient mice which provided a notable resistance against acute infection caused by *T. gondii* (Fachado et al., 2003). During in-*vitro* study, tachyzoites of *T. gondii* were effectively killed when rIFN-γ was injected into mice. Such data recommend that rIFN-γ might be operative for toxoplasmosis therapy within immunosuppressed individuals whose T cell function is impaired. Though therapy which is immune-based, chiefly via exogenous IFN-γ administration, is an auspicious way to treat such infectious diseases still it is overwhelmed by important issues like side effects. In addition, higher prices make it unfeasible for larger-scale usage within developing nations.

### 3.4. Immunotherapy to Tackle Viral Opportunistic Infections

*Cytomegalovirus* and *Human Polyomavirus*-2 (also known as JC virus) are known to cause progressive multifocal leukoencephalopathy (PML). *Human herpesvirus*-8 (also known as Kaposi sarcoma-associated herpesvirus) is an opportunistic virus. Different immunotherapies and immunomodulation are mentioned here which could use to tackle opportunistic infections caused by viruses.

*3.4.1. Modifying Innate Mechanisms to Target Viral Infections*
Here the physical-chemical barrier, the first line of defense, is provided by innate immunity against infections. Microbe-associated molecular patterns are recognized by Toll-like receptors (TLRs). TLRs sense invasive microbes and they are part of innate mechanisms (Kumar et al., 2009). Signals are transduced by TLRs so that cells could reply through activating antiviral and proinflammatory processes. TLR 3, 7, 8 and 9 sense the viral species and

medications. TLRs un-specifically enhance the TLR-facilitated responses and possess the capability of working in numerous viral infections.

Some of the agonists of TLRs such as ANA245, CPG-10101 and isatoribine are effective against infections caused by HCV (McHutchison et al., 2006). Imiquimod, an agonist of TLR7, is clinically approved for treating exterior anogenital warts produced by human *papillomavirus* (HPV). Whereas its efficiency within lesions produced by HCV, *Molluscum contagiosum* virus, and Herpes simplex virus is debatable (Miller et al., 2008). The influenza virus is suppressed by compound 3M-011, which is an agonist of TLR8 and TLR7 (Hammerbeck et al., 2007). There is an extreme need for further elaborate studies to be conducted in the zone of enhancing innate immunity against infections caused by viruses.

### *3.4.2. CAR T-Cell Immunotherapy*

A recently approved immunotherapeutic approach involves enhancing T-cell function through a chimeric antigen receptor (CAR). CAR-T-cells are engineered to express a recombinant receptor, usually incorporating a T-cell specificity determining antibody derivative binding to a specific receptor expressed on targeted cells fused to a transmembrane signaling domain, thus allowing MHC-independent T-cell activation. CAR T-cell therapy is a form of adoptive cell therapy, which involves isolating a patient's peripheral blood T-cells and modifying it to express a CAR ex-vivo followed by administering the CAR-T-cells to the patient. As many first-generation CARs were anergic, subsequent modifications allowed engineering of not only targeting and transmembrane signaling domains such as a CD3 chain but also by incorporation of a co-stimulatory receptor-like CD28.

The third and fourth-generation CARs were developed with the addition of a second co-stimulatory molecule and an inducible gene to express proinflammatory or pro-proliferative cytokines, respectively. Some of the very first CAR T-cells developed for HIV envelope protein (Env)-targeted treatment were generated by replacing the extracellular T cell receptor domain with CD4 (CD4-CAR). While the CAR treatment was safe and feasible in clinical trials, it failed to reduce viral load permanently (Seif et al., 2019). Second-generation CARs containing an intracellular CD28 domain exhibited higher cytokine production and better control over HIV replication in-vitro. Both strategies rendered the CD4-CARs resistant to infection and provided persistent control of infection in animal models. Novel second-generation CARs targeting the HIV CD4 binding site or glycoprotein 120 (gp120) antigens were designed based on single-chain variable fragments derived from

Env-specific bNAbs. These CARs have demonstrated specific killing of HIV-infected cells, but their antiviral efficacy was highly variable and strain-dependent. This was improved by combining second-generation glycan CARs, targeting variable glycans regions on the surface of HIV with CCR5 ablation, enabling superior control of viral replication over the CAR alone. First-generation anti-gp120 CARs, efficiently stimulated activation, and cytokine secretion mediating lysis of Env-expressing HIV-1 infected CD4 T-cells in vitro.

The third-generation gp120-specific CARs had superior lysis over CD4 CARs and remained uninfected upon interaction with the cell-free virus. Furthermore, the CAR-induced cytolysis of reactivated HIV reservoirs isolated from infected patients. The main drawback of this approach is the mutants viral escape which renders the therapy inefficient. To improve treatment efficacy, bi- and tri-specific CARs targeting up to three HIV antigens were designed. Two bi-specific CARs comprising a CD4 domain fused to gp120 or a carbohydrate recognition domain C-type human lectin that binds to conserved glycans on Env showed superior suppressive activity compared to CD4-CAR (Niessl et al., 2020). Recently, CAR T-cells with three functionally distinct HIV Env-binding domains were engineered to express two distinct CARs on the same T-cell or one CAR with two targeting elements. Targets included gp120 CD4 binding site, a CD4- induced gp120 epitope, and a C46 peptide or C34-CXCR4 (Maldini et al., 2020).

C46 peptide and C34-CXCR4 inhibit viral fusion thereby preventing infection of the CAR T-cell. Bi- and tri-specific CARs were able to prevent HIV infection of the CARs while efficiently killing other HIV-positive cells in humanized mouse models (Ali et al., 2020). There are currently two human clinical trials trying to eradicate the latent HIV reservoir; one is a bNAb-based CAR T-cell therapy (NCT03240328); while the other is a CD4- CAR T-cell therapy in conjunction with CCR5 ablation (NCT03617198). In addition to HIV, two cytomegaloviruses (CMV)- specific CARs have recently been described. One CAR, based on a 21E9 glycoprotein subunit H targeting antibody, has superior activity in all functional tests. Surprisingly, it had 10-fold less binding affinity compared to other CARs targeting the same protein suggesting affinity not to be the main determinant of effectiveness. The 21E9-CAR, however, binds to a unique epitope suggested being more accessible. While the CAR showed only modest CD8+ T-cell killing of CMV-infected cells it provided support as a potential candidate for immunotherapy of CMV since it also stimulated cytokine release, the proliferation of effectors and the suppression of viral replication (Maldini et al., 2020).

### 3.4.3. Use of Cytokines

In immunotherapy of HIV, a significant role is played by cytokines application. Initially, it was dreaded that IL-2 might raise the cell pool of host for the viral species, nonetheless, this seems to be predominated via the impact of IL-2 in increasing CD8+ T-cell-facilitated viral suppression. IL-2 may mediate its effect through the induction of IL-7, expression of CD25 on CD4+ T cells, as well as proliferation and survival of CD4+, CD8+, and NK cells. Low-dose or long-term intermittent use of IL-2 has been shown to have clinical benefits in some cases (Durier et al., 2007), and may aid in therapeutic immunization of chronically infected patients. However, IL-2 treatment was found to not stimulate CD8+ T cell proliferation or be useful in other cases, and the actual impact on clinical outcome is still debatable (Smith et al., 2007). IL-7, the thymopoietic cytokine, can renew T cells without increasing viral load in macaques, and granulocyte colony-stimulating factor (G-CSF) can increase CD4+ T cell progenitors and improve CD4+ T cell counts (Beq et al., 2006). IL-12 and IL-15 potentiate CD8+ T cell effector and memory responses elicited by DNA vaccines against SIV, and control the virus in-*vivo*. IFN-γ administration or co-expression with SIV candidates elicits a Th1 response and produces a remarkable effect on plasma viral load and CD4+ T cell counts in monkeys (Kaneyasu et al., 2005).

### 3.4.4. Dendritic Cell Therapy

In treating HIV infection, dendritic cell therapy has gained importance. Dendritic cells expressing Nef targeted to either lysosomes or cytoplasm using mRNA-transfections could be ex-vivo applied for expanding anti-HIV CD4+ T cells and CD8+ (Kavanagh et al., 2006). Dendritic cells pulsed with inactivated SIV or HIV persuade precise and vigorous Th1 responses which distinctly lead to reduced viral load within the plasma. In infected persons, particular immune responses are stimulated by RNA-electroporated mature dendritic cells or autologous antigen (inactivated virus or peptide)-pulsed which results in viral load reduction (Mason et al., 2009).

When dendritic cells are used so they can harness the pathways related to antigen presentation. Dendritic cells are a particular type of cells that could do antigen presentation by both MHC-II and MHC-I pathways and direct antigens to specific compartments. They can expand antigen-particular CD8+ T cells or CD4+ cells both in-*vitro* and in-*vivo*. Another treatment intervention comprising immune cells (CD34+ or CD4+) has been established against HIV, comprising "autologous gene-modified T cells" for treating the virus which is resistant to the drug within advanced AIDS stages (Cohen 2007).

## Conclusion

Opportunistic infections by parasites, fungi, viruses and bacteria are a major health issues. Great economic losses occur because of the increasing quantity of invasive medical interventions and immunosuppressive therapies in conjunction with raising resistance to fungal, parasitic, bacterial, and viral strains. In addition, there are limitations of traditional anti-parasitic, antifungal, anti-bacterial, and anti-viral chemotherapeutic agents. It is a great challenge to treat opportunistic infections. Consequently, for treating opportunistic infections caused by different microorganisms, immunotherapy and immunomodulation are interesting strategies. In current decades, advancements have been made in the usage of present anti-parasitic, antiviral, antifungal, and antibacterial immunotherapies. Strategies for tackling opportunistic infections through enhancing the immunity of the host comprise the usage of regulatory and effector cells in addition to the usage of growth factors, recombinant cytokines, abs, granulocyte and granulocyte-macrophage CSF. Novel approaches to tackle opportunistic infections in immuno-suppressive hosts target signaling pathways within the cells through smaller molecular inhibitors such as checkpoint inhibitors. These checkpoint inhibitors have not only shown substantial efficiency within cancer therapy but also have shown their antifungal effect in early infection caused by *Aspergillus*. Hence, checkpoint inhibitors turn out to be a hopeful innovative immunotherapeutic choice for treating opportunistic infections.

## References

Abt, M. C., Lewis, B. B., Caballero, S., Xiong, H., Carter, R. A., Sušac, B., ... & Pamer, E. G. (2015). Innate immune defenses mediated by two ILC subsets are critical for protection against acute Clostridium difficile infection. *Cell Host & Microbe*, *18*(1), 27-37.

Ackermann, M., Kempf, H., Hetzel, M., Hesse, C., Hashtchin, A. R., Brinkert, K., ... &Lachmann, N. (2018). Bioreactor-based mass production of human iPSC-derived macrophages enables immunotherapies against bacterial airway infections. *Nature Communications*, *9*(1), 1-13.

Ali, A., Chiuppesi, F., Nguyen, M., Hausner, M. A., Nguyen, J., Kha, M., ... & Yang, O. O. (2020). Chimeric antigen receptors targeting human cytomegalovirus. *The Journal of Infectious Diseases*, *222*(5), 853-862.

Ali, S. O., Yu, X. Q., Robbie, G. J., Wu, Y., Shoemaker, K., Yu, L., ... & Jafri, H. S. (2019). Phase 1 study of MEDI3902, an investigational anti–Pseudomonas aeruginosa PcrV and Psl bispecific human monoclonal antibody, in healthy adults. *Clinical Microbiology and Infection, 25*(5), 629-e1.

Almeida, F., Rodrigues, M. L., & Coelho, C. (2019). The still underestimated problem of fungal diseases worldwide. *Frontiers in Microbiology, 10*, 214.

Ang, A. L., & Linn, Y. C. (2011). Treatment of severe neutropenic sepsis with granulocyte transfusion in the current era–experience from an adult haematology unit in Singapore. *Transfusion Medicine, 21*(1), 13-24.

Bacher, P., Jochheim-Richter, A., Mockel-Tenbrink, N., Kniemeyer, O., Wingenfeld, E., Alex, R., ... &Scheffold, A. (2015). Clinical-scale isolation of the total Aspergillus fumigatus–reactive T–helper cell repertoire for adoptive transfer. *Cytotherapy, 17*(10), 1396-1405.

Beq, S., Nugeyre, M. T., Fang, R. H. T., Gautier, D., Legrand, R., Schmitt, N., ... &Israël, N. (2006). IL-7 induces immunological improvement in SIV-infected rhesus macaques under antiviral therapy. *The Journal of Immunology, 176*(2), 914-922.

Bozza, S., Gaziano, R., Lipford, G. B., Montagnoli, C., Bacci, A., Di Francesco, P., ... & Romani, L. (2002). Vaccination of mice against invasive aspergillosis with recombinant Aspergillus proteins and CpG oligodeoxynucleotides as adjuvants. *Microbes and Infection, 4*(13), 1281-1290.

Bozza, S., Perruccio, K., Montagnoli, C., Gaziano, R., Bellocchio, S., Burchielli, E., ... & Romani, L. (2003). A dendritic cell vaccine against invasive aspergillosis in allogeneic hematopoietic transplantation. *Blood, 102*(10), 3807-3814.

Brenner, D. J., Steigerwalt, A. G., &McDade, J. E. (1979). Classification of the Legionnaires' disease bacterium: Legionella pneumophila, genus novum, species nova, of the family Legionellaceae, familia nova. *Annals of Internal Medicine, 90*(4), 656-658.

Brown, G. D. (2011). Innate antifungal immunity: the key role of phagocytes. *Annual Review of Immunology, 29*, 1-21.

Brown, G. D., Denning, D. W., Gow, N. A., Levitz, S. M., Netea, M. G., & White, T. C. (2012). Hidden killers: human fungal infections. *Science Translational Medicine, 4*(165), 165rv13-165rv13.

Buddhisa, S., Rinchai, D., Ato, M., Bancroft, G. J., &Lertmemongkolchai, G. (2015). Programmed death ligand 1 on Burkholderia pseudomallei–infected human polymorphonuclear neutrophils impairs T cell functions. *The Journal of Immunology, 194*(9), 4413-4421.

Buddingh, E. P., Leentjens, J., van der Lugt, J., Dik, W. A., Gresnigt, M. S., Netea, M. G., ... & Driessen, G. J. (2015). Interferon-gamma immunotherapy in a patient with refractory disseminated candidiasis. *The Pediatric Infectious Disease Journal, 34*(12), 1391-1394.

Campos, A. B., Ribeiro, J., Boutolleau, D., & Sousa, H. (2016). Human cytomegalovirus antiviral drug resistance in hematopoietic stem cell transplantation: current state of the art. *Reviews in Medical Virology, 26*(3), 161-182.

Casadevall, A., & Pirofski, L. A. (2012). Immunoglobulins in defense, pathogenesis, and therapy of fungal diseases. *Cell Host & Microbe, 11*(5), 447-456.

Chen, K., Huang, J., Gong, W., Iribarren, P., Dunlop, N. M., & Wang, J. M. (2007). Toll-like receptors in inflammation, infection and cancer. *International Immunopharmacology*, *7*(10), 1271-1285.

Chen, T. K., Groncy, P. K., Javahery, R., Chai, R. Y., Nagpala, P., Finkelman, M., ... &Walsh, T. J. (2016). Successful treatment of Aspergillus ventriculitis through voriconazole adaptive pharmacotherapy, immunomodulation, and therapeutic monitoring of cerebrospinal fluid (1→ 3)-β-d-glucan. *Sabouraudia*, *55*(1), 109-117.

Chen, X. M., O'Hara, S. P., Nelson, J. B., Splinter, P. L., Small, A. J., Tietz, P. S., ... & LaRusso, N. F. (2005). Multiple TLRs are expressed in human cholangiocytes and mediate host epithelial defense responses to Cryptosporidium parvum via activation of NF-κB. *The Journal of Immunology*, *175*(11), 7447-7456.

Chuang, Y. M., He, L., Pinn, M. L., Tsai, Y. C., Cheng, M. A., Farmer, E., ... & Hung, C. F. (2021). Albumin fusion with granulocyte-macrophage colony-stimulating factor acts as an immunotherapy against chronic tuberculosis. *Cellular & Molecular Immunology*, *18*(10), 2393-2401.

Cohen, J. (2007). Building an HIV-proof immune system. *Science*, *317*(5838), 612-614.

Corzo-León, D. E., Satlin, M. J., Soave, R., Shore, T. B., Schuetz, A. N., Jacobs, S. E., & Walsh, T. J. (2015). Epidemiology and outcomes of invasive fungal infections in allogeneic haematopoietic stem cell transplant recipients in the era of antifungal prophylaxis: a single-centre study with focus on emerging pathogens. *Mycoses*, *58*(6), 325-336.

D'Alessio, F. R., Tsushima, K., Aggarwal, N. R., West, E. E., Willett, M. H., Britos, M. F., ... & King, L. S. (2009). CD4+ CD25+ Foxp3+ Tregs resolve experimental lung injury in mice and are present in humans with acute lung injury. *The Journal of Clinical Investigation*, *119*(10), 2898-2913.

da Fonseca-Martins, A. M., Ramos, T. D., Pratti, J. E., Firmino-Cruz, L., Gomes, D. C. O., Soong, L., ... & de Matos Guedes, H. L. (2019). Immunotherapy using anti-PD-1 and anti-PD-L1 in Leishmaniaamazonensis-infected BALB/c mice reduce parasite load. *Scientific Reports*, *9*(1), 1-13.

Das, M., Zhu, C., &Kuchroo, V. K. (2017). Tim-3 and its role in regulating anti-tumor immunity. *Immunological reviews*, *276*(1), 97-111.

Das, S., Suarez, G., Beswick, E. J., Sierra, J. C., Graham, D. Y., & Reyes, V. E. (2006). Expression of B7-H1 on gastric epithelial cells: its potential role in regulating T cells during Helicobacter pylori infection. *The Journal of Immunology*, *176*(5), 3000-3009.

Davies, S. I., &Muranski, P. (2017). T cell therapies for human polyomavirus diseases. *Cytotherapy*, *19*(11), 1302-1316.

Delsing, C. E., Gresnigt, M. S., Leentjens, J., Preijers, F., Frager, F. A., Kox, M., ... &Netea, M. G. (2014). Interferon-gamma as adjunctive immunotherapy for invasive fungal infections: a case series. *BMC Infectious Diseases*, *14*(1), 1-12.

Doring, G., Conway, S. P., Heijerman, H. G., Hodson, M. E., Hoiby, N., Smyth, A., &Touw, D. J. (2000). Antibiotic therapy against Pseudomonas aeruginosa in cystic fibrosis: a European consensus. *European Respiratory Journal*, *16*(4), 749-767.

Driscoll, J. A., Brody, S. L., &Kollef, M. H. (2007). The epidemiology, pathogenesis and treatment of Pseudomonas aeruginosa infections. *Drugs*, *67*(3), 351-368.

Dromer, F. R. A. N. Q. O. I. S. E., Charreire, J., Contrepois, A., Carbon, C., & Yeni, P. (1987). Protection of mice against experimental cryptococcosis by anti-Cryptococcus neoformans monoclonal antibody. *Infection and Immunity*, *55*(3), 749-752.

Durier, C., Capitant, C., Lascaux, A. S., Goujard, C., Oksenhendler, E., Poizot-Martin, I., ... & Lévy, Y. (2007). Long-term effects of intermittent interleukin-2 therapy in chronic HIV-infected patients (ANRS 048–079 Trials). *Aids*, *21*(14), 1887-1897.

Elphick, G. F., Querbes, W., Jordan, J. A., Gee, G. V., Eash, S., Manley, K., ... & Atwood, W. J. (2004). The human polyomavirus, JCV, uses serotonin receptors to infect cells. *Science*, *306*(5700), 1380-1383.

Fachado, A., Rodriguez, A., Angel, S. O., Pinto, D. C., Vila, I., Acosta, A., ... &Lannes-Vieira, J. (2003). Protective effect of a naked DNA vaccine cocktail against lethal toxoplasmosis in mice. *Vaccine*, *21*(13-14), 1327-1335.

Feigman, M. S., Kim, S., Pidgeon, S. E., Yu, Y., Ongwae, G. M., Patel, D. S., ... & Pires, M. M. (2018). Synthetic immunotherapeutics against Gram-negative pathogens. *Cell Chemical Biology*, *25*(10), 1185-1194.

Flanigan, T., Whalen, C., Turner, J., Soave, R., Toerner, J., Havlir, D., & Kotler, D. (1992). Cryptosporidium infection and CD4 counts. *Annals of Internal Medicine*, *116*(10), 840-842.

Gigliotti, F., & Hughes, W. T. (1988). Passive immunoprophylaxis with specific monoclonal antibody confers partial protection against Pneumocystis carinii pneumonitis in animal models. *The Journal of Clinical Investigation*, *81*(6), 1666-1668.

Gong, J. H., Zhang, M., Modlin, R. L., Linsley, P. S., Iyer, D., Lin, Y., & Barnes, P. F. (1996). Interleukin-10 downregulates Mycobacterium tuberculosis-induced Th1 responses and CTLA-4 expression. *Infection and Immunity*, *64*(3), 913-918.

Gooley, T. A., Chien, J. W., Pergam, S. A., Hingorani, S., Sorror, M. L., Boeckh, M., ... & McDonald, G. B. (2010). Reduced mortality after allogeneic hematopoietic-cell transplantation. *New England Journal of Medicine*, *363*(22), 2091-2101.

Hammerbeck, D. M., Burleson, G. R., Schuller, C. J., Vasilakos, J. P., Tomai, M., Egging, E., ... & Miller, R. L. (2007). Administration of a dual toll-like receptor 7 and toll-like receptor 8 agonist protects against influenza in rats. *Antiviral Research*, *73*(1), 1-11.

Hendrickson, J. A., Hu, C., Aitken, S. L., & Beyda, N. (2019). Antifungal resistance: a concerning trend for the present and future. *Current Infectious Disease Reports*, *21*(12), 1-8.

Holokai, L., Chakrabarti, J., Broda, T., Chang, J., Hawkins, J. A., Sundaram, N., ... &Zavros, Y. (2019). Increased programmed death-ligand 1 is an early epithelial cell response to Helicobacter pylori infection. *PLoS Pathogens*, *15*(1), e1007468.

Hubbell, J. A., Thomas, S. N., & Swartz, M. A. (2009). Materials engineering for immunomodulation. *Nature*, *462*(7272), 449-460.

Imaculada Muniz-Junqueira, M. (2007). Immunomodulatory therapy associated to anti-parasite drugs as a way to prevent severe forms of malaria. *Current Clinical Pharmacology*, *2*(1), 59-73.

Jarvis, J. N., Meintjes, G., Rebe, K., Williams, G. N., Bicanic, T., Williams, A., ... & Harrison, T. S. (2012). Adjunctive interferon-γ immunotherapy for the treatment of

HIV-associated cryptococcal meningitis: a randomized controlled trial. *AIDS (London, England)*, *26*(9), 1105.

Jayaraman, P., Jacques, M. K., Zhu, C., Steblenko, K. M., Stowell, B. L., Madi, A., ... & Behar, S. M. (2016). TIM3 mediates T cell exhaustion during Mycobacterium tuberculosis infection. *PLoS Pathogens*, *12*(3), e1005490.

Kalinina, A. A., Nesterenko, L. N., Bruter, A. V., Balunets, D. V., Chudakov, D. M., Izraelson, M., ... &Kazansky, D. B. (2020). Adoptive immunotherapy based on chain-centric TCRs in treatment of infectious diseases. *Iscience*, *23*(12), 101854.

Kaneyasu, K., Kita, M., Ohkura, S., Yamamoto, T., Ibuki, K., Enose, Y., ... & Hayami, M. (2005). Protective Efficacy of Nonpathogenic Nef-Deleted SHIV Vaccination Combined with Recombinant IFN-γ Administration against a Pathogenic SHIV Challenge in Rhesus Monkeys. *Microbiology and Immunology*, *49*(12), 1083-1094.

Karwa, R., &Wargo, K. A. (2009). Efungumab: a novel agent in the treatment of invasive candidiasis. *Annals of Pharmacotherapy*, *43*(11), 1818-1823.

Kavanagh, D. G., Kaufmann, D. E., Sunderji, S., Frahm, N., Le Gall, S., Boczkowski, D., ... & Bhardwaj, N. (2006). Expansion of HIV-specific CD4+ and CD8+ T cells by dendritic cells transfected with mRNA encoding cytoplasm-or lysosome-targeted Nef. *Blood*, *107*(5), 1963-1969.

Ketelut-Carneiro, N., Silva, G. K., Rocha, F. A., Milanezi, C. M., Cavalcanti-Neto, F. F., Zamboni, D. S., & Silva, J. S. (2015). IL-18 triggered by the Nlrp3 inflammasome induces host innate resistance in a pulmonary model of fungal infection. *The Journal of Immunology*, *194*(9), 4507-4517.

Kumar, H., Kawai, T., & Akira, S. (2009). Pathogen recognition in the innate immune response. *Biochemical Journal*, *420*(1), 1-16.

Kunzmann, V., Kimmel, B., Herrmann, T., Einsele, H., & Wilhelm, M. (2009). Inhibition of phosphoantigen-mediated γδ T-cell proliferation by CD4+ CD25+ FoxP3+ regulatory T cells. *Immunology*, *126*(2), 256-267.

La Manna, M. P., Orlando, V., Tamburini, B., Badami, G. D., Dieli, F., &Caccamo, N. (2020). Harnessing unconventional T cells for immunotherapy of tuberculosis. *Frontiers in Immunology*, *11*, 2107.

Langan, E. A., Graetz, V., Allerheiligen, J., Zillikens, D., Rupp, J., &Terheyden, P. (2020). Immune checkpoint inhibitors and tuberculosis: an old disease in a new context. *The Lancet Oncology*, *21*(1), e55-e65.

Larsen, R. A., Pappas, P. G., Perfect, J., Aberg, J. A., Casadevall, A., Cloud, G. A., ... &Dismukes, W. E. (2005). Phase I evaluation of the safety and pharmacokinetics of murine-derived anticryptococcal antibody 18B7 in subjects with treated cryptococcal meningitis. *Antimicrobial Agents and Chemotherapy*, *49*(3), 952-958.

Latgé, J. P. (1999). Aspergillus fumigatus and aspergillosis. *Clinical Microbiology Reviews*, *12*(2), 310-350.

Lauruschkat, C. D., Einsele, H., & Loeffler, J. (2018). Immunomodulation as a therapy for Aspergillus infection: current status and future perspectives. *Journal of Fungi*, *4*(4), 137.

Lessa, F. C., Gould, C. V., & McDonald, L. C. (2012). Current status of Clostridium difficile infection epidemiology. *Clinical Infectious Diseases*, *55*(suppl_2), S65-S70.

Lu, L. L., Chung, A. W., Rosebrock, T. R., Ghebremichael, M., Yu, W. H., Grace, P. S., ... & Alter, G. (2016). A functional role for antibodies in tuberculosis. *Cell*, *167*(2), 433-443.

Ludwig, E., Bonanni, P., Rohde, G., Sayiner, A., & Torres, A. (2012). The remaining challenges of pneumococcal disease in adults. *European Respiratory Review*, *21*(123), 57-65.

Luster, A. D., Alon, R., & von Andrian, U. H. (2005). Immune cell migration in inflammation: present and future therapeutic targets. *Nature Immunology*, *6*(12), 1182-1190.

MacGregor, P., Gonzalez-Munoz, A. L., Jobe, F., Taylor, M. C., Rust, S., Sandercock, A. M., ... & Carrington, M. (2019). A single dose of antibody-drug conjugate cures a stage 1 model of African trypanosomiasis. *PLoS Neglected Tropical Diseases*, *13*(5), e0007373.

Mahmoud, Y. A. G., El-Naggar, M. E., Abdel-Megeed, A., & El-Newehy, M. H. (2021). Recent Advancements in Microbial Polysaccharides: Synthesis and Applications. *Polymers*, *13*(23), 4136.

Maldini, C. R., Claiborne, D. T., Okawa, K., Chen, T., Dopkin, D. L., Shan, X., ... & Allen, T. M. (2020). Dual CD4-based CAR T cells with distinct costimulatory domains mitigate HIV pathogenesis in vivo. *Nature Medicine*, *26*(11), 1776-1787.

Martin, J. N., Ganem, D. E., Osmond, D. H., Page-Shafer, K. A., Macrae, D., &Kedes, D. H. (1998). Sexual transmission and the natural history of human herpesvirus 8 infection. *New England Journal of Medicine*, *338*(14), 948-954.

Masihi, K. N. (2000). Immunomodulators in infectious diseases: panoply of possibilites. *International Journal of Immunopharmacology*, *22*(12), 1083-1091.

Mason, R. D., Alcantara, S., Peut, V., Loh, L., Lifson, J. D., De Rose, R., & Kent, S. J. (2009). Inactivated simian immunodeficiency virus-pulsed autologous fresh blood cells as an immunotherapy strategy. *Journal of Virology*, *83*(3), 1501-1510.

McCarthy, M. W., Denning, D. W., & Walsh, T. J. (2017). Future research priorities in fungal resistance. *The Journal of Infectious Diseases*, *216*(suppl_3), S484-S492.

McHutchison, J. G., Bacon, B. R., Gordon, S. C., Lawitz, E., Shiffman, M., Afdhal, N. H., ... & Davis, H. L. (2006). 111 Final results of a multi-center phase 1b, randomized, placebo-controlled, doseescalation trial of CPG 10101 in patients with chronic hepatitis C virus. *Journal of Hepatology*, (44), S49.

Medici, N. P., & Del Poeta, M. (2015). New insights on the development of fungal vaccines: from immunity to recent challenges. *Memorias do Instituto Oswaldo Cruz*, *110*, 966-973.

Mehrad, B., Strieter, R. M., &Standiford, T. J. (1999). Role of TNF-α in pulmonary host defense in murine invasive aspergillosis. *The Journal of Immunology*, *162*(3), 1633-1640.

Mellinghoff, S. C., von Bergwelt-Baildon, M., Schößer, H. A., &Cornely, O. A. (2019). A novel approach to candidemia? The potential role of checkpoint inhibition. *Medical Mycology*, *57*(2), 151-154.

Micheletti, F., Monini, P., Fortini, C., Rimessi, P., Bazzaro, M., Andreoni, M., ... &Gavioli, R. (2002). Identification of cytotoxic T lymphocyte epitopes of human herpes virus 8. *Immunology*, *106*(3), 395-403.

Miller, R. L., Meng, T. C., &Tomai, M. A. (2008). The antiviral activity of Toll-like receptor 7 and 7/8 agonists. *Drug News & Perspectives, 21*(2), 69-87.

Mor, V., Rella, A., Farnoud, A. M., Singh, A., Munshi, M., Bryan, A., ... & Del Poeta, M. (2015). Identification of a new class of antifungals targeting the synthesis of fungal sphingolipids. *MBio, 6*(3), e00647-15.

Motley, M. P., Banerjee, K., & Fries, B. C. (2019). Monoclonal antibody-based therapies for bacterial infections. *Current Opinion on Infectious Diseases, 32*(3), 210.

Murray, H. W. (1994). Interferon-gamma and host antimicrobial defense: current and future clinical applications. *The American Journal of Medicine, 97*(5), 459-467.

Nagai, H., Guo, J., Choi, H., &Kurup, V. (1995). Interferon-γ and tumor necrosis factor-α protect mice from invasive aspergillosis. *Journal of Infectious Diseases, 172*(6), 1554-1560.

Naran, K., Nundalall, T., Chetty, S., & Barth, S. (2018). Principles of immunotherapy: implications for treatment strategies in cancer and infectious diseases. *Frontiers in Microbiology, 9*, 3158.

Neofytos, D., Horn, D., Anaissie, E., Steinbach, W., Olyaei, A., Fishman, J., ... & Marr, K. (2009). Epidemiology and outcome of invasive fungal infection in adult hematopoietic stem cell transplant recipients: analysis of Multicenter Prospective Antifungal Therapy (PATH) Alliance registry. *Clinical Infectious Diseases, 48*(3), 265-273.

Niessl, J., Baxter, A. E., Mendoza, P., Jankovic, M., Cohen, Y. Z., Butler, A. L., ... & Kaufmann, D. E. (2020). Combination anti-HIV-1 antibody therapy is associated with increased virus-specific T cell immunity. *Nature Medicine, 26*(2), 222-227.

Okazaki, T., & Wang, J. (2005). PD-1/PD-L pathway and autoimmunity. *Autoimmunity, 38*(5), 353-357.

Pachl, J., Svoboda, P., Jacobs, F., Vandewoude, K., van der Hoven, B., Spronk, P., ... &Mycograb Invasive Candidiasis Study Group. (2006). A randomized, blinded, multicenter trial of lipid-associated amphotericin B alone versus in combination with an antibody-based inhibitor of heat shock protein 90 in patients with invasive candidiasis. *Clinical Infectious Diseases, 42*(10), 1404-1413.

Papaioannou, N. E., Beniata, O. V., Vitsos, P., Tsitsilonis, O., & Samara, P. (2016). Harnessing the immune system to improve cancer therapy. *Annals of Translational Medicine, 4*(14).

Peck, M., Rothenberg, M. E., Deng, R., Lewin-Koh, N., She, G., Kamath, A. V., ... &Tavel, J. A. (2019). A phase 1, randomized, single-ascending-dose study to investigate the safety, tolerability, and pharmacokinetics of DSTA4637S, an anti-Staphylococcus aureusthiomab antibody-antibiotic conjugate, in healthy volunteers. *Antimicrobial Agents and Chemotherapy, 63*(6), e02588-18.

Pedersen, F. K., Johansen, K. S., Rosenkvist, J., Tygstrup, L., &Valerius, N. H. (1979). Refractory Pneumocystis carinii infection in chronic granulomatous disease: successful treatment with granulocytes. *Pediatrics, 64*(6), 935-938.

Perfect, J. R. (2016). Is there an emerging need for new antifungals?. *Expert Opinion on Emerging Drugs, 21*(2), 129-131.

Perruccio, K., Tosti, A., Burchielli, E., Topini, F., Ruggeri, L., Carotti, A., ... & Velardi, A. (2005). Transferring functional immune responses to pathogens after haploidentical hematopoietic transplantation. *Blood, 106*(13), 4397-4406.

Pflughoeft, K. J., & Versalovic, J. (2012). Human microbiome in health and disease. *Annual Review of Pathology: Mechanisms of Disease, 7,* 99-122.

Pirofski, L. A., & Casadevall, A. (2015). What is infectiveness and how is it involved in infection and immunity?. *BMC Immunology, 16*(1), 1-6.

Prajeeth, C. K., Haeberlein, S., Sebald, H., Schleicher, U., & Bogdan, C. (2011). Leishmania-infected macrophages are targets of NK cell-derived cytokines but not of NK cell cytotoxicity. *Infection and Immunity, 79*(7), 2699-2708.

Putignani, L., &Menichella, D. (2010). Global distribution, public health and clinical impact of the protozoan pathogen Cryptosporidium. *Interdisciplinary Perspectives on Infectious Diseases, 2010.*

Que, Y. A., Lazar, H., Wolff, M., François, B., Laterre, P. F., Mercier, E., ... &Eggimann, P. (2014). Assessment of panobacumab as adjunctive immunotherapy for the treatment of nosocomial Pseudomonas aeruginosa pneumonia. *European Journal of Clinical Microbiology & Infectious Diseases, 33*(10), 1861-1867.

Quezada, G., Koshkina, N. V., Zweidler-McKay, P., Zhou, Z., Kontoyiannis, D. P., &Kleinerman, E. S. (2008). Intranasal granulocyte-macrophage colony-stimulating factor reduces the Aspergillus burden in an immunosuppressed murine model of pulmonary aspergillosis. *Antimicrobial Agents and Chemotherapy, 52*(2), 716-718.

Ramirez-Ortiz, Z. G., & Means, T. K. (2012). The role of dendritic cells in the innate recognition of pathogenic fungi (A. fumigatus, C. neoformans and C. albicans). *Virulence, 3*(7), 635-646.

Riggs, M. W. (2002). Recent advances in cryptosporidiosis: the immune response. *Microbes and Infection, 4*(10), 1067-1080.

Riley RS, June CH, Langer R et al. (2019). Delivery technologies for cancer immunotherapy. *Nat Rev Drug Discov,* 18, 175– 96.

Roilides, E., Blake, C., Holmes, A., Pizzo, P. A., & Walsh, T. J. (1996). Granulocyte-macrophage colony-stimulating factor and interferon-γ prevent dexamethasone-induced immunosuppression of antifungal monocyte activity against Aspergillus fumigatus hyphae. *Journal of Medical and Veterinary Mycology, 34*(1), 63-69.

Roilides, E., Lamaignere, C. G., &Farmaki, E. (2002). Cytokines in immunodeficient patients with invasive fungal infections: an emerging therapy. *International Journal of Infectious Diseases, 6*(3), 154-163.

Roy RM and Klein BS. (2012) Dendritic cells in antifungal immunity and vaccine design. *Cell Host Microbe,* 11, 436–446.

Safdar, A., Rodriguez, G., Ohmagari, N., Kontoyiannis, D. P., Rolston, K. V., Raad, I. I., & Champlin, R. E. (2005). The safety of interferon-γ-1b therapy for invasive fungal infections after hematopoietic stem cell transplantation. *Cancer, 103*(4), 731-739.

Safdar, A., Rodriguez, G., Zuniga, J., Al Akhrass, F., Georgescu, G., & Pande, A. (2013). Granulocyte macrophage colony-stimulating factor in 66 patients with myeloid or lymphoid neoplasms and recipients of hematopoietic stem cell transplantation with invasive fungal disease. *Actahaematologica, 129*(1), 26-34.

Schmidt, S., Tramsen, L., Hanisch, M., Latgé, J. P., Huenecke, S., Koehl, U., &Lehrnbecher, T. (2011). Human natural killer cells exhibit direct activity against Aspergillus fumigatus hyphae, but not against resting conidia. *Journal of Infectious Diseases, 203*(3), 430-435.

Schmidt, S., Tramsen, L., Perkhofer, S., Lass-Flörl, C., Hanisch, M., Röger, F., ... &Lehrnbecher, T. (2013). Rhizopus oryzae hyphae are damaged by human natural killer (NK) cells, but suppress NK cell mediated immunity. *Immunobiology, 218*(7), 939-944.

Schneider, A., Blatzer, M., Posch, W., Schubert, R., Lass-Flörl, C., Schmidt, S., &Lehrnbecher, T. (2016). Aspergillus fumigatus responds to natural killer (NK) cells with upregulation of stress related genes and inhibits the immunoregulatory function of NK cells. *Oncotarget, 7*(44), 71062.

Scriven, J. E., Tenforde, M. W., Levitz, S. M., & Jarvis, J. N. (2017). Modulating host immune responses to fight invasive fungal infections. *Current Opinion in Microbiology, 40*, 95-103.

See, J. X., Chandramathi, S., Abdulla, M. A., Vadivelu, J., & Shankar, E. M. (2017). Persistent infection due to a small-colony variant of Burkholderia pseudomallei leads to PD-1 upregulation on circulating immune cells and mononuclear infiltration in viscera of experimental BALB/c mice. *PLoS Neglected Tropical Diseases, 11*(8), e0005702.

Seif, M., Einsele, H., & Löffler, J. (2019). CAR T cells beyond cancer: hope for immunomodulatory therapy of infectious diseases. *Frontiers in Immunology, 10*, 2711.

Shao, C., Qu, J., He, L., Zhang, Y., Wang, J., Zhou, H., ... & Liu, X. (2005). Dendritic cells transduced with an adenovirus vector encoding interleukin-12 are a potent vaccine for invasive pulmonary aspergillosis. *Genes & Immunity, 6*(2), 103-114.

Shen, B., Qian, A., Lao, W., Li, W., Chen, X., Zhang, B., ... & Sun, Y. (2019). Relationship between Helicobacter pylori and expression of programmed death-1 and its ligand in gastric intraepithelial neoplasia and early-stage gastric cancer. *Cancer Management and Research, 11*, 3909.

Silva, R. A., Pais, T. F., &Appelberg, R. (1998). Evaluation of IL-12 in immunotherapy and vaccine design in experimental Mycobacterium avium infections. *The Journal of Immunology, 161*(10), 5578-5585.

Sionov, E., Mendlovic, S., & Segal, E. (2005). Experimental systemic murine aspergillosis: treatment with polyene and caspofungin combination and G-CSF. *Journal of Antimicrobial Chemotherapy, 56*(3), 594-597.

Smith, K. A., Andjelic, S., Popmihajlov, Z., Kelly-Rossini, L., Sass, A., Lesser, M., ... & Bellman, P. (2007). Immunotherapy with canarypox vaccine and interleukin-2 for HIV-1 infection: termination of a randomized trial. *PLoS Clinical Trials, 2*(1), e5.

Stephen-Victor, E., Karnam, A., Fontaine, T., Beauvais, A., Das, M., Hegde, P., ... &Bayry, J. (2017). Aspergillus fumigatus cell wall α-(1, 3)-glucan stimulates regulatory T-cell polarization by inducing PD-L1 expression on human dendritic cells. *The Journal of Infectious Diseases, 216*(10), 1281-1294.

Stevenson, M. M., Su, Z., Sam, H., & Mohan, K. (2001). Modulation of host responses to blood-stage malaria by interleukin-12: from therapyto adjuvant activity. *Microbes and Infection, 3*(1), 49-59.

Stuehler, C., Kuenzli, E., Jaeger, V. K., Baettig, V., Ferracin, F., Rajacic, Z., ... & Khanna, N. (2015). Immune reconstitution after allogeneic hematopoietic stem cell transplantation and association with occurrence and outcome of invasive aspergillosis. *The Journal of Infectious Diseases, 212*(6), 959-967.

Styczynski, J., Czyzewski, K., Wysocki, M., Gryniewicz-Kwiatkowska, O., Kolodziejczyk-Gietka, A., Salamonowicz, M., ... & Gil, L. (2016). Increased risk of infections and infection-related mortality in children undergoing haematopoietic stem cell transplantation compared to conventional anticancer therapy: a multicentre nationwide study. *Clinical Microbiology and Infection, 22*(2), 179-e1.

Susa, M., Ticac, B., Rukavina, T., Doric, M., &Marre, R. (1998). Legionella pneumophila infection in intratracheally inoculated T cell-depleted or-nondepleted A/J mice. *The Journal of Immunology, 160*(1), 316-321.

Suurs, F. V., Lub-de Hooge, M. N., de Vries, E. G., & de Groot, D. J. A. (2019). A review of bispecific antibodies and antibody constructs in oncology and clinical challenges. *Pharmacology & Therapeutics, 201*, 103-119.

Szabo, S. J., Kim, S. T., Costa, G. L., Zhang, X., Fathman, C. G., &Glimcher, L. H. (2000). A novel transcription factor, T-bet, directs Th1 lineage commitment. *Cell, 100*(6), 655-669.

Tacke, R., Sun, J., Uchiyama, S., Polovina, A., Nguyen, D. G., &Nizet, V. (2019). Protection against lethal multidrug-resistant bacterial infections using macrophage cell therapy. *Infectious Microbes & Diseases, 1*(2), 61-69.

Teixeira, L. K., Fonseca, B. P., Barboza, B. A., & Viola, J. P. (2005). The role of interferon-gamma on immune and allergic responses. *Memórias do Instituto Oswaldo Cruz, 100*, 137-144.

Tormo, N., Solano, C., Benet, I., Nieto, J., De La Camara, R., Lopez, J., ... & Navarro, D. (2011). Reconstitution of CMV pp65 and IE-1-specific IFN-γ CD8+ and CD4+ T-cell responses affording protection from CMV DNAemia following allogeneic hematopoietic SCT. *Bone Marrow Transplantation, 46*(11), 1437-1443.

Torosantucci, A., Chiani, P., Bromuro, C., De Bernardis, F., Palma, A. S., Liu, Y., ... & Cassone, A. (2009). Protection by anti-β-glucan antibodies is associated with restricted β-1, 3 glucan binding specificity and inhibition of fungal growth and adherence. *PloS One, 4*(4), e5392.

Triantafyllou, E., Gudd, C. L., Mawhin, M. A., Husbyn, H. C., Trovato, F. M., Siggins, M. K., ... &Thursz, M. R. (2021). PD-1 blockade improves Kupffer cell bacterial clearance in acute liver injury. *The Journal of Clinical Investigation, 131*(4).

Unsinger, J., Burnham, C. A. D., McDonough, J., Morre, M., Prakash, P. S., Caldwell, C. C., ... & Hotchkiss, R. S. (2012). Interleukin-7 ameliorates immune dysfunction and improves survival in a 2-hit model of fungal sepsis. *The Journal of Infectious Diseases, 206*(4), 606-616.

van de Berg, P. J., van Leeuwen, E. M., Ten Berge, I. J., & van Lier, R. (2008). Cytotoxic human CD4+ T cells. *Current Opinion in Immunology, 20*(3), 339-343.

Voigt, J., Hünniger, K., Bouzani, M., Jacobsen, I. D., Barz, D., Hube, B., ... &Kurzai, O. (2014). Human natural killer cells acting as phagocytes against Candida albicans and mounting an inflammatory response that modulates neutrophil antifungal activity. *The Journal of Infectious Diseases, 209*(4), 616-626.

Wan, L., Zhang, Y., Lai, Y., Jiang, M., Song, Y., Zhou, J., ... & Wang, C. (2015). Effect of granulocyte-macrophage colony-stimulating factor on prevention and treatment of invasive fungal disease in recipients of allogeneic stem-cell transplantation: a prospective multicenter randomized phase IV trial. *Journal of Clinical Oncology*, *33*(34), 3999-4006.

Wang, F., Hou, H., Wu, S., Tang, Q., Huang, M., Yin, B., ... & Sun, Z. (2015). Tim-3 pathway affects NK cell impairment in patients with active tuberculosis. *Cytokine*, *76*(2), 270-279.

Wang, Z., Li, G., Dou, S., Zhang, Y., Liu, Y., Zhang, J., ... & Han, G. (2020). Tim-3 promotes listeria monocytogenes immune evasion by suppressing major histocompatibility complex class I. *The Journal of Infectious Diseases*, *221*(5), 830-840.

West, K. A., Gea-Banacloche, J., Stroncek, D., & Kadri, S. S. (2017). Granulocyte transfusions in the management of invasive fungal infections. *British Journal of Haematology*, *177*(3), 357-374.

White, P. L., Posso, R. B., & Barnes, R. A. (2015). Analytical and clinical evaluation of the PathoNosticsAsperGenius assay for detection of invasive aspergillosis and resistance to azole antifungal drugs during testing of serum samples. *Journal of Clinical Microbiology*, *53*(7), 2115-2121.

Wright, C. R., Ward, A. C., & Russell, A. P. (2017). Granulocyte colony-stimulating factor and its potential application for skeletal muscle repair and regeneration. *Mediators of Inflammation*, *2017*.

Wüthrich, M., DeepeJr, G. S., & Klein, B. (2012). Adaptive immunity to fungi. *Annual Review of Immunology*, *30*, 115-148.

Wykes, M. N., & Lewin, S. R. (2018). Immune checkpoint blockade in infectious diseases. *Nature Reviews Immunology*, *18*(2), 91-104.

Xin, H., Dziadek, S., Bundle, D. R., & Cutler, J. E. (2008). Synthetic glycopeptide vaccines combining β-mannan and peptide epitopes induce protection against candidiasis. *Proceedings of the National Academy of Sciences*, *105*(36), 13526-13531.

## Chapter 4

# Genetically Engineered Bacteriophages for the Treatment of ESKAPE Pathogens

### Haseesh Rahithya Nandam[1], Anjali Parmar[1,2], Krithikashri Sarathy[1] and Sutharsan Govindarajan[1,*]

[1]Department of Biological sciences,
SRM University AP, Amaravati, India
[2]School of Biotechnology,
Amrita Vishwa Vidyapeetham, Amritapuri, Kerala, India

## Abstract

Bacterial infections have an enormous impact on public health, which are combated using antibiotics. The World Health Organization has predicted that drug-resistant disease caused by continuous use of antibiotics could cause nearly 10 million deaths each year by 2050 and catastrophic damage to the economy. With no successful discovery of novel set of antibiotics for nearly four decades, antimicrobial resistance has become a serious public health threat. As human race is already facing a dramatic challenge due to resistance in this antibiotic era, there is an urgent need for alternative therapies to combat this issue. That said, phage therapy – which uses bacterial viruses (phages) to combat bacterial infections and has been around for more than 100 years – is considered a promising alternative to antibiotic therapy, especially against multidrug-resistant pathogens. Phage therapy has several advantages over antibiotic therapy: high specificity, i.e., targeting a specific pathogen but not the rest of the microbiome; ability to overcome bacterial biofilms; and ability

---

*Corresponding Author's Email: sutharsan.g@srmap.edu.in.

In: Interdisciplinary Approaches on Opportunistic Infections …
Editors: Jayapradha Ramakrishnan and Ganesh Babu Malli Mohan
ISBN: 978-1-68507-984-0
© 2022 Nova Science Publishers, Inc.

to deliver novel antimicrobials like CRISPR-Cas nucleases. However, despite holding several advantages, conventional phage therapy technology is not widely successful. In this chapter, we highlight how bacteriophages are used to treat infections caused by pathogens, especially ESKAPE pathogens. We also summarize the currently available methods for bacteriophage genome engineering and discuss the advantages of using genetically engineered bacteriophages over conventional methods to combat bacterial infections.

## 1. Introduction to Phage Therapy

Bacteriophages are viruses that specifically infect, parasitize, and kill bacteria. Although bacteriophages have been used to treat bacterial infections since their discovery by Frederick Twort and Felix d'Hérelle, (d'Herelle, 1961; Twort, 1961; Sulakvelidze, Alavidze and Morris Jr, 2001), their therapeutic potential fell out of favor with the advent of antibiotics. In medical history, antibiotic therapy is considered one of the most effective and successful therapeutic interventions. However, extensive and continuous use of antibiotics has led to rapid emergence of multidrug-resistant (MDR) bacteria, thereby garnering increased interest in alternative therapies. That said, phage therapy has recently gained enormous attention as an alternative therapy for bacterial infections (Gordillo Altamirano and Barr, 2019; Kortright et al., 2019). Bacteriophages are biological entities abundantly present in the environment and, therefore, they can be easily isolated and propagated in large volumes. Bacteriophages exhibit high specificity and are highly evolved species and, therefore, they infect only specific bacterial strains or species and not the normal microbiota of the host (Sulakvelidze, Alavidze and Morris Jr, 2001); however, a few bacteriophages can infect across the genera. Furthermore, bacteriophages propagate only at the site of infection, are self-limiting and self-dosing, and do not persist when their specific bacterial pathogen becomes absent. However, identification of effective and exact phages against the target pathogen is difficult, which is a major limitation of phage therapy.

### 1.1. Bacteriophage Infection

Phage infection is a step-wise process. First, phages attach to the surface of the host cell by binding to specific bacterial surface proteins or cell wall components followed by the injection of their genetic material into the host cell. Upon injection of their DNA or RNA into the host cell, the phage adopts one of the following two replication strategies—lytic or lysogenic cycle. In lytic cycle, once a bacteriophage enters the host cell, it redirects the bacterial/host synthetic machinery to produce more viral genomes and proteins. The newly synthesized bacteriophage particles are then assembled and packed followed by cell lysis, which releases new virions that find and infect other neighboring host cells. In lysogenic cycle, the phage genomes are integrated into the bacterial chromosome or are maintained as non-integrated episomes. Under unfavorable conditions, the prophages, that is phage DNAs, are excised out and undergo lytic cycle and eventually release phage virions (Stern and Sorek, 2011)Duckworth and Gulig, 2002). Because of their ability to kill specific bacteria and not integrate into the host genome, lytic bacteriophages are majorly used in phage therapy (Sulakvelidze, Alavidze and Morris Jr, 2001).

Phage therapy has become a common practice in Eastern Europe and the Soviet Union and, currently, it constitutes a standard medical practice in the Republic of Georgia (Silva et al., 2021). Despite its efficacy, phage therapy is still not adopted as a standard practice in the West due to several reasons: lack of specific regulatory framework, availability of little or no data on safety, need for customized patient-tailored phage cocktail, and need to conduct large-scale *in vivo* studies on the efficacy and safety of standardized phage products (Moelling, Broecker and Willy, 2018). As Fleming predicted in his Nobel lecture in 1945, an increase in MDR bacterial infections and a decline in the discovery of novel antibiotics led to a renewed interest in phage therapy in the West. Recent antimicrobial studies have proved that bacteria that cause nosocomial and community-acquired infections have become pan-drug resistant, which is alarming and a clinical threat to humans (Sulis et al., 2022). Each step of antibiotic development is challenged by the emerging microbial resistance. Antibiotic resistance is mostly acquired by alteration of target genes or acquisition of plasmids encoding resistance genes. These encoded genes produce lytic enzymes, change membrane permeability, alter efflux action, and escape from the action of antibiotics (Frieri, Kumar and Boutin, 2017). Therefore, a multidisciplinary, collaborative, and regulatory approach is needed for combating antimicrobial resistance. Although several alternative treatment options like stem cell-anti microbial peptides, probiotics, and nanobiotics are available (Kumar et al., 2021), the usage of bacteriophages against MDR pathogens appears to be widely successful and easier to implement compared to other approaches (Sulakvelidze, Alavidze and Morris Jr, 2001).

## 1.2. ESKAPE Pathogens and Phage Therapy

In 2017, WHO published a list of antibiotic-resistant "priority pathogens" that included a group of bacteria referred to as ESKAPE pathogens: *Enterococcus faecium, Staphylococcus aureus, Klebsiella pneumoniae, Acinetobacter baumannii, Pseudomonas aeruginosa*, and *Enterobacter* species (Shrivastava, Shrivastava and Ramasamy, 2018). ESKAPE pathogens represent new paradigms in pathogenesis, transmission, and resistance and are often resistant to one or more antibiotics (Rice, 2010; De Oliveira et al., 2020). As they are resistant to multiple drugs and spread rapidly through hospital-acquired infections, they are considered a major threat to human health (Shrivastava, Shrivastava and Ramasamy, 2018)(Mulani et al., 2019). In the following sections, we briefly describe the individual ESKAPE pathogen and the phage therapy effective against them.

### *1.2.1. Enterococcus faecium*

*Enterococcus faecium* is a gram-positive, facultative, anaerobic, and opportunistic pathogen. Enterococcus spp. comprise nearly 35 species and they typically inhabit the gastrointestinal tract (GIT). Nearly 90% of bacterial isolates recovered from endocarditis, bacteremia, urinary tract infections, meningitis, and root canal infections are associated with *E. faecium*. *E. faecium* is absolutely resistant to ampicillin, β-lactam antibiotics, and imipenem and intrinsically resistant to clindamycin (a lincosamide), quinupristin (class B streptogramin) and dalfopristin (class A streptogramin), and vancomycin (Klare et al., 2003; van Hal et al., 2021). Previous studies have shown the efficacy of phage therapy against *E. faecium* infections (Gao, Howden and Stinear, 2018). In a recent study, a cocktail of two *E. faecium* bacteriophages namely EFgrKN and EFgrNG was used to successfully treat *E. faecium* infection in a 1-year-old child following a third liver transplant at the University Medical Center Hamburg—Eppendorf in 2019 (Paul et al., 2021). Similarly, EFDG1 *E. faecium* phage was also used to treat persistent *E. faecium* infections of root canals. Nearly, a 7-log reduction of bacterial leakage in root apex was observed when an ex vivo two-chamber bacterial leakage model of human teeth was subjected to EFDG1 phage treatment (Khalifa et al., 2015). In a study by Tinoco et al., (2016)., extracted human dentin root segments were cemented into a sealable double chamber and inoculated for 7 days, with an overnight suspension of either VR *E. faecalis* V583 or *E. faecalis* JH2-2, which is sensitive to vancomycin but resistant to fusidic acid and rifampin. These phages effectively eliminated the drug resistant pathogens (Tinoco et al., 2016). Another study showed an 18% reduction for JH2-2-infected models and a 99% reduction for V583-infected models when treated with genetically engineered phage phiEf11/phiFL1C(Δ36)PnisA (Bolocan et al., 2019). The above studies prove the efficacy of phage therapy in the treatment of root canal and other infections.

### *1.2.2. Staphylococcus aureus*

*S. aureus* is a gram-positive, opportunistic pathogen and is the leading pathogen responsible for deaths caused by antimicrobial resistance and nosocomial infections (Thwaites et al., 2011; Cong, Yang and Rao, 2020). This member of firmicutes is often found on upper respiratory tracts and skin and causes minor skin infection, food poisoning, pneumonia, bacteremia, sepsis, endocarditis, etc. *S. aureus* is capable of forming multispecies biofilm on implanted medical devices and human body and, therefore, is frequently associated with wound infections post-surgery. It is resistant to β-lactams, aminoglycoside, β-lactamase-resistant penicillins (methicillin), vancomycin, and so on (Lowy, 2003). In particular, methicillin-resistant *S. aureus* (MRSA) has become a major public health threat as infections caused by them are difficult to treat (Lee et al., 2018). That said, bacteriophages are emerging as viable alternatives for the treatment of drug-resistant *S. aureus* infections (Azam and Tanji, 2019). Of note, a phase I clinical trial on bacteriophage cocktail AB-SAO1 (Sa83+Sa87+J-Sa36) was recently carried out in patients with chronic rhinosinusitis (Patil, Banerji, Kanojiya, Koratkar, et al., 2021). The study found the intranasal administration of AB-SAO1 to be safe and as an alternative to antibiotics. Similarly, intranasal administration of bacteriophage cocktail AB-SAO1 in a mouse model of acute pneumonia decreased the clinical counts of *S. aureus* isolates by 94-95%. A previous study by Fish et al. (2016) showed that treatment of diabetic toe ulcers with SB-1 phage prevented amputation and healed wounds; moreover, no recurrence of infection occurred (Fish et al., 2016). In addition, *S. aureus* phages UPMK_1 and UPMK_2, due to the presence of lytic enzymes, exhibited a high biofilm-degrading ability against MRSA infection (Dakheel et al., 2022).

### 1.2.3. Klebsiella pneumoniae

*K. pneumoniae* isa gram-negative pathogen that belongs to Enterobacteriaceae family. It is the most prevalent pathogen that causes both hospital- and community-acquired infections and, therefore, is a mounting pathological threat to humans. It causes a wide range of diseases including pneumonias; infections of the urinary tract, lower biliary tract, upper respiratory tract, and surgical wound sites; inflammatory diseases such as thrombophlebitis, cholecystitis, osteomyelitis, and meningitis; diarrhea; bacteremia; and sepsis. It is frequently resistant to aminoglycosides, fluoroquinolones, tetracyclines, chloramphenicol, and trimethoprim and beta-lactam antibiotics, except carbapenems (Victor et al., 2007; De Rosa et al., 2015). Infections with carbapenem-resistant Enterobacteriaceae or carbapenemase-producing Enterobacteriaceae are emerging as important challenges in healthcare settings (Dakheel et al., 2022). Various studies have examined the efficacy of phage therapy against this pathogen. A previous study analyzed the biofilm-eliminating capacity of bacteriophage TSK1 on *K. pneumoniae* biofilm developed *in vitro* and found that the TSK1 degraded the capsular polysaccharides present in the biofilm by producing a depolymerase enzyme (Tabassum et al., 2018). Similarly, treatment of MDR *K. pneumoniae* KP/01 with bacteriophage ZCKP1 when applied at a high multiplicity of infection (50 PFU/CFU) showed greater than 50% reduction in bacterial counts and biofilm biomass (Tabassum et al., 2018; Taha et al., 2018).

### 1.2.4. Acinetobacter baumannii

*A. baumannii* is a gram-negative, non-motile, and non-fermentative bacillus that is resistant to almost all first-line drugs (Peleg, Seifert and Paterson, 2008; Kyriakidis et al., 2021). It is the major causative agent of nosocomial disease and infects the urinary tract, lungs, or any wound site. *A. baumannii* is colloquially referred to as "Iraqibacter" due to its sudden emergence in the treatment facilities during the Iraq War. *A. baumannii* strains producing carbapenemase carrying imipenem metallo-β-lactamases are resistant to both colistin and imipenem antibiotics and these strains can evade most traditional antimicrobials (Peleg, Seifert and Paterson, 2008; Lee et al., 2017;Kyriakidis et al., 2021). Several studies have successfully used bacteriophages against *A. baumannii*. For example, PlyF307 was shown to significantly reduce planktonic and biofilm of *A. baumannii* both *in vitro* and *in vivo* (Lood et al., 2015). Furthermore, a cocktail of φIVB was shown to be effective in the treatment of pancreatic pseudocyst infection caused by *A. baumannii* in a diabetic patient (Schooley et al., 2017). Another recent study showed that, in a mouse model, bacteriophages ΦFG02 and ΦCO01 were effective against clinical isolates of *A. baumannii*, and phage-resistant mutants were found to be sensitive to antibiotics (Gordillo Altamirano et al., 2021).

### 1.2.5. Pseudomonas aeruginosa

*P. aeruginosa* is a gram-negative bacillus and is one of the major opportunistic pathogens that plays a significant role in nosocomial, acute, and chronic infections. It exhibits innate resistance to beta-lactams, aminoglycosides, carbapenems, cephalosporins, monobactams, and fluoroquinolones (Hancock and Speert, 2000; Lambert, 2002; Gellatly and Hancock, 2013) and, therefore, nosocomial infections associated with this organism including gastrointestinal infection, urinary tract infections, and blood stream infection are difficult to treat. *P. aeruginosa* is a major pathogen extensively studied for phage therapy. For example, the first controlled clinical trial performed in 2019 proved the efficacy of phage cocktail preparation on chronic otitis caused by antibiotic-resistant *P. aeruginosa* (Wright et al., 2009). Another study found that *P. aeruginosa* phages δ and 001A inhibited bacterial growth and biofilm formation significantly at all MOIs, but σ-1 phage significantly inhibited bacterial growth only at very high MOIs (Knezevic et al., 2011). In 2011, a 26-year-old cystic fibrosis patient infected with two strains of MDR *P. aeruginosa* was treated with AP-PA01, a cocktail of four bacteriophages produced by AmpliPhi Biosciences Corporation. The results showed that the cocktail effectively eliminated *P. aeruginosa* colonies (Kay et al., 2011). Another study by Tümmler (2019) showed that a combination of phage Podoviridae LUZ7 and streptomycin effectively killed *P. aeruginosa*. Furthermore, researchers were able to restore antibiotic sensitivity in MDR *P. aeruginosa* with a single application of lytic phage OMKO1, which utilizes the multidrug efflux systems such as MexAB and MexXY receptors (Chan et al., 2016).

## 1.3. Limitations of Phage Therapy

The current data available on phage therapy are scarce and conflicting and the trials were not performed according to global clinical standards; therefore, no consensus has yet been reached regarding the treatment of bacterial infections using phage therapy. Few major limitations encountered during phage therapy are described in the following sections.

*Identification of Therapeutic Bacteriophages:* Identification of suitable bacteriophages for therapeutic purpose is still a daunting, complicated, and time-consuming task. Although a large number of bacteriophages have been isolated and are available against a pathogen, identifying the specific bacteriophage for a given pathogen is immediately not possible. Moreover, the host specificity of a bacteriophage has to be demonstrated before considering it a potential therapeutic agent. This is a relatively complicated process since the lytic capacity of a bacteriophage can change according to the experimental procedure, dose, and delivery method (Loc-Carrillo and Abedon, 2011; Nilsson, 2019). Furthermore, it is more important to ensure that the therapeutic bacteriophage genome does not contain integrase genes such as in the lysogenic type, antibiotic-resistant genes, genes for phage-encoded toxins, or genes for other bacterial virulence factors. Thus, despite the availability of a specific bacteriophage against a pathogen, the presence of an annotated sequenced genome limits the ability of a phage to be used as a therapeutic agent (Loc-Carrillo and Abedon, 2011; Henein, 2013; Nilsson, 2019).

*Polymicrobial Infections:* ESKAPE pathogens as well as other pathogens are capable of causing polymicrobial infections in patients (Patil, Banerji, Kanojiya and Saroj, 2021). In such cases, phage therapy becomes obsolete if it is targeted against only one pathogen, and administration of antibiotics becomes the highly recommended treatment option. Therefore, understanding the status of polymicrobial infection in a patient becomes more important before attempting phage therapy. Researchers and clinicians have previously used phage cocktails capable of infecting two different bacterial pathogens (Nir-Paz *et al.*, 2019). Thus, increasing the diversity of phages in cocktails increases the chances of success of phage therapy, but comes with an additional burden of understanding the polymicrobial infectivity status of the patient.

*Formulation and Stabilization of Phage Pharmaceutical:* Generally, bacteriophages are used as formulations and not as solutions. The advantages of having bacteriophages in the form of formulations are two-fold – prolonged shelf life and increased sustained release. However, the shelf life of bacteriophages is still poor, and therefore less stable, compared to antibiotics. This restricts the pharmaceutical industries from being able to commercially produce bacteriophages for therapeutic purposes (Nilsson, 2019).

## 1.4. Genetic Engineering of Bacteriophages

Phage therapy using natural phages may be limited due to rapid selection of phage resistant bacteria, enhanced immunogenicity due to prolonged treatment. Phages do not induce resistance in the host and do not show cross-resistance to antibiotics; these characteristics make them highly effective against MDR bacteria and biofilms. However, they can cause phage resistance in bacterial host, which becomes a major obstacle in the process of developing effective phage therapy. Some resistance mechanisms include loss or mutation of the bacterial receptor that results in blockage of phage adsorption and horizontal acquisition of a restriction-modification system or development of CRISPR-mediated adaptive immunity. These mechanisms result in the degradation of the injected phage DNA. Furthermore, use of lytic phages can also be alarming as the rapid lysis of a large number of bacteria *in vivo* may release endotoxins and superantigens that may induce an inflammatory response. Moreover, immunogenicity along with its clinical consequence *in vivo* is a concern as well. These problems could be overcome by using genetically engineered phages, which seem to be promising (Bárdy et al., 2016; Chen et al., 2019). In the following sections, we summarize the currently available methods of phage genome engineering and their advantages.

### *1.4.1. Homologous Recombination*

Homologous recombination (HR) is one of the methods most commonly used to engineer phage genomes (Lenneman et al., 2021). In bacterial hosts, HR can occur between two homologous DNA sequences, which can start from 23 bp. However, the rates of recombination tend to be higher when longer homologous DNA sequences that are more than 100 bp are used (Pines et al., 2015). HR is a naturally occurring phenomenon and is exploited by genetic engineering methods to produce random or designed recombinant phages. Various phage genome modifications including gene insertions, replacements, or deletions similar to the bacterial counterparts can be done by HR. In the process of HR, the target gene is first cloned into a plasmid that has two regions of homology with the phage genome. The homologous regions determine the region in the phage genome where the foreign gene will be incorporated. The host with the donor plasmid is then infected by the phage to be engineered, after which HR takes place between the plasmid and the phage genome, with the heterologous gene being integrated into the phage genome. Since the recombination frequencies are usually very lowranging from $10^{10}$ to $10^4$, isolation of a modified phage becomes a tedious process. However, recombinant phages can be easily selected by introducing marker genes such as beta-galactosidase, luciferase, green fluorescent protein (GFP), and other phage-specific marker genes (Pires et al., 2016). A recent study has used anti-CRISPRs as phage-specific marker to identify recombinant phages (Mayo-Muñoz et al., 2018). Positive selection (fluorescence markers) and negative selection (CRISPR-Cas9 targeted against the wild-type phage) can also be used to select engineered phage particles.

### 1.4.2. Genome Rebooting and Rebuilding

Genome rebooting and rebuilding are novel, synthetic biology strategies that use DNA fragments assembled *in vitro* for engineering phage genomes in the bacterial host. In this method, small- to medium-sized DNA fragments are assembled into complete full-length phage genomes through either transformation-associated recombination (TAR) or *in vitro* enzymatic assembly (Gibson assembly). These methods enable the engineering of fully synthetic phage genomes and make the introduction of mutations, deletions, or insertions at any genomic region of interest in the phage genome relatively easy. A previous study has shown that cell-free approach, which is independent of transformation efficiency, provides the ability to work with gene sequences that encode products that are toxic to intermediate strains used for cloning (Shin, Jardine and Noireaux, 2012). These methods are suitable for genome engineering of phages that infect gram-negative bacteria; however, polyethylene glycol-mediated genome transformation allows the rebooting of recombinant phages in gram-positive bacteria. In genome rebooting, assembled genomic DNAs are reactivated inside a suitable host cell or in cell-free systems, whereas in genome rebuilding, DNA segments are grouped with the help of restriction sites, which allow the alteration of DNA in each section without affecting the other sections. Previously, a chimeric T7 phage genome was synthesized using this approach and it was possible to generate a viable T7 recombinant (Shin, Jardine and Noireaux, 2012; Pires et al., 2016). Both genome rebooting and rebuilding methods are capable of generating recombinant phages with assembled DNA fragments. However, sequencing information of other phages of interest is highly important for designing DNA fragments for these methods.

### 1.4.3. Bacteriophage Recombineering of Electroporated DNA (BRED)

BRED technique uses heterologous recombination proteins to promote phage DNA recombination (Marinelli et al., 2008; Payaslian, Gradaschi and Piuri, 2021). This method was initially employed to modify mycobacteriophages

(Marinelli et al., 2008), but later on has been used to modify phages that target various bacterial hosts. BRED technique is suitable for various phage genome modifications including deletion, insertion, and replacement of genes, and creation of point mutations. In this method, recombineering substrates, i.e., phage DNA and dsDNA, are coelectroporated into electro-competent bacterial cells carrying a plasmid that encodes proteins promoting high levels of HR. dsDNA substrate comprises the DNA fragments to be inserted within the regions of homology to the loci immediately upstream and downstream of the region of the phage genome to be modified. After electroporation, the bacterial cells are recovered, mixed with wild-type bacterial host, and plated. The plates are then checked for the presence of phage plaques. Individual plaques, indicative of bacterial cell lysis, are then screened by PCR for the correctly mutated phage genome. By using this method, phages are modified at high frequencies (10 to 15%), thus enabling competent mutants to be screened by PCRs. However, this technique requires highly competent bacterial hosts (Marinelli et al., 2008; Pines et al., 2015; Payaslian, Gradaschi and Piuri, 2021), which is a major disadvantage.

### *1.4.4. CRISPR-Cas-Mediated Genome Engineering*

This system has become a versatile genome-editing technology extensively used for engineering the genomes of various organisms including bacteirophages (Martel and Moineau, 2014). Studies have shown that CRISPR along with *Cas* genes forms an adaptive immune system in bacteria and Archaea (Amitai and Sorek, 2016). Kiro et al. described a method to efficiently engineer T7 phage genome by using type I-E CRISPR-Cas system (Kiro, Shitrit and Qimron, 2014). This method utilizes the HR pathway and selects recombinants in the presence of target-specific Cas nuclease. First, HR was used as a template to delete a nonessential T7 gene (gene 1.7). The T7 phage was propagated in a bacterial host carrying a plasmid with homologous regions to the upstream and downstream of the interested phage gene 1.7, enabling the deletion of the gene 1.7. To further propagate the desired recombinant phages, a CRISPR-based counter-selection system was used. The type I-E CRISPR-Cas system was designed to cleave all the non-recombinant phage genomes, which contained the original gene 1.7, but not the recombinant phage genomes, which lacked gene 1.7. Thus, only the recombinant phages were enriched. A major advantage of this method is the direct screening of recombinant phages from a large pool of wild-type phages. Similarly, the *Streptococcus thermophilus* type II-A CRISPR-Cas system was used to select Streptococcus phage 2972 recombinants that underwent point mutations, small and large DNA deletions, and gene replacements (Martel and Moineau, 2014).

### 1.4.5. Yeast-Based Assembly of Phage Genomes

Generally, propagation of phage genomes in a bacterial host can be toxic for the host, which is a major limitation that restricts the growth of recombinant phages. To overcome this issue, researchers employed *Saccharomyces cerevisiae*, a heterologous host, as a model yeast to assemble and grow recombinant phages (Jaschke et al., 2012; Rita Costa et al., 2018). Of note, homologous recombination is particularly effective in *S. cerevisiae*, and phage genomes do not cause toxicity in yeast and can be maintained stably. This method utilizes a *S. cerevisiae*-bacterial shuttle vector cloned with the gene of interest along with overhangs homologous to the ends of the phage genome. The recombinant phage genomes thus produced are extracted from the yeast and introduced into the bacteria for further selection and growth (Jaschke et al., 2012; Pires et al., 2016; Rita Costa et al., 2018).

## 2. Future Prospects

The focus on phage therapy has dramatically increased since the emergence of antibiotic resistance. Currently, it is being recognized as an ideal strategy to combat the threats of antibiotic resistance posed by ESKAPE and other pathogens. However, although phage therapy presents numerous advantages such as possibility of isolation of numerous bacteriophages against clinical pathogens, *in vitro* and *in vivo* evaluation of antibacterial efficacy, and capability of immune tolerance, multiple limitations still exist that restrict envisioning phage therapy as a widely accepted treatment strategy. Creating awareness, conducting standard clinical trials, and rapidly improvising the required technologies are the need of the hour to make phage therapy a standard medical practice. Moreover, governments should implement standard regulatory policies regarding phage therapy, which will help clinicians adopt phage therapy as a treatment procedure against antibiotic-resistant pathogens. Development of genetically modified bacteriophages, development of broad host range phages, phages with less propensity of gene transfer, and phages capable of delivering novel antimicrobials like CRISPR-Cas nucleases are the major advantages of phage therapy on multiple fronts. However, future studies are needed to explore their potential side effects and to derive standard ethics policies before utilizing bacteriophages as therapeutic agents.

## Acknowledgments

We thank members of the Sutharsan Govindarajan lab at SRM University – AP for helpful discussions. S.G acknowledges support from DST-SERB Core Research Grant (CRG/2020/003295).

## References

Amitai, G. and Sorek, R. (2016) 'CRISPR–Cas adaptation: insights into the mechanism of action,' *Nature Reviews Microbiology*, 14(2), pp. 67–76.

Azam, A. H. and Tanji, Y. (2019) 'Peculiarities of Staphylococcus aureus phages and their possible application in phage therapy,' *Applied Microbiology and Biotechnology*, 103(11), pp. 4279–4289.

Bárdy, P., Pantůček, R., Benešík, M., & Doškař, J. (2016). 'Genetically modified bacteriophages in applied microbiology,' *Journal of Applied Microbiology*, 121(3), pp. 618–633.

Bolocan, Upadrasta, Bettio, Clooney, Draper, Ross, & Hill. (2019). 'Evaluation of phage therapy in the context of Enterococcus faecalis and its associated diseases,' *Viruses*, 11(4), p. 366.

Chan, B. K., Sistrom, M., Wertz, J. E., Kortright, K. E., Narayan, D., & Turner, P. E. (2016). 'Phage selection restores antibiotic sensitivity in MDR Pseudomonas aeruginosa,' *Scientific Reports*, 6(1), pp. 1–8.

Chen, Y., Batra, H., Dong, J., Chen, C., Rao, V. B., & Tao, P. (2019). 'Genetic engineering of bacteriophages against infectious diseases,' *Frontiers in Microbiology*, 10, p. 954.

Cong, Y., Yang, S. and Rao, X. (2020) 'Vancomycin resistant Staphylococcus aureus infections: A review of case updating and clinical features,' *Journal of Advanced Research*, 21, pp. 169–176.

Dakheel, Khulood Hamid, Raha Abdul Rahim, Jameel R. Al-Obaidi, Vasantha Kumari Neela, Tan Geok Hun, Mohd Noor Mat Isa, Nurhanani Razali, and Khatijah Yusoff. (2022) 'Proteomic analysis revealed the biofilm-degradation abilities of the bacteriophage UPMK_1 and UPMK_2 against Methicillin-resistant Staphylococcus aureus,' *Biotechnology Letters*, pp. 1–10.

De Oliveira, David M. P., Brian M. Forde, Timothy J. Kidd, Patrick N. A. Harris, Mark A. Schembri, Scott A. Beatson, David L. Paterson, and Mark J. Walker. (2020) 'Antimicrobial resistance in ESKAPE pathogens,' *Clinical microbiology reviews*, 33(3), pp. e00181-19.

De Rosa, Francesco G, Silvia Corcione, Rossana Cavallo, Giovanni Di Perri, and Matteo Bassetti. (2015) 'Critical issues for Klebsiella pneumoniae KPC-carbapenemase producing K. pneumoniae infections: a critical agenda,' *Future Microbiology*, 10(2), pp. 283–294.

d'Herelle, M. F. (1961) 'Sur un microbe invisible antagoniste des bacilles dysentériques [*On an invisible microbe antagonist of dysenteric bacilli*],' *Acta Kravsi*.

Duckworth, D. H. and Gulig, P. A. (2002) 'Bacteriophages,' *BioDrugs*, 16(1), pp. 57–62.

Fish, R., E. Kutter, G. Wheat, B. Blasdel, M. Kutateladze, and S. Kuhl. (2016) 'Bacteriophage treatment of intransigent diabetic toe ulcers: a case series,' *Journal of Wound Care*, 25(Sup3), pp. S27–S33.

Frieri, M., Kumar, K. and Boutin, A. (2017) 'Antibiotic resistance,' *Journal of Infection and Public Health*, 10(4), pp. 369–378.

Gao, W., Howden, B. P. and Stinear, T. P. (2018) 'Evolution of virulence in Enterococcus faecium, a hospital-adapted opportunistic pathogen,' *Current Opinion in Microbiology*, 41, pp. 76–82.

Gellatly, S. L. and Hancock, R. E. W. (2013) 'Pseudomonas aeruginosa: new insights into pathogenesis and host defenses,' *Pathogens and Disease*, 67(3), pp. 159–173.

Gordillo Altamirano, F. L. and Barr, J. J. (2019) 'Phage therapy in the postantibiotic era,' *Clinical Microbiology Reviews*, 32(2), pp. e00066-18.

Gordillo Altamirano, F. L., Forsyth, J. H., Patwa, R., Kostoulias, X., Trim, M., Subedi, D., Archer, S. K., Morris, F. C., Oliveira, C., Kielty, L., Korneev, D., O'Bryan, M. K., Lithgow, T. J., Peleg, A. Y., & Barr, J. J. (2021) 'Bacteriophage-resistant Acinetobacter baumannii are resensitized to antimicrobials,' *Nature Microbiology*, 6(2), pp. 157–161.

Hancock, R. E. W. and Speert, D. P. (2000) 'Antibiotic resistance in Pseudomonas aeruginosa: mechanisms and impact on treatment,' *Drug Resistance Updates*, 3(4), pp. 247–255.

Henein, A. (2013) 'What are the limitations on the wider therapeutic use of phage?,' *Bacteriophage*, 3(2), p. e24872.

Jaschke, Paul R., Erica K. Lieberman, Jon Rodriguez, Adrian Sierra, and Drew Endy. (2012) 'A fully decompressed synthetic bacteriophage øX174 genome assembled and archived in yeast,' *Virology*, 434(2), pp. 278–284.

Kay, M. K., Thomas C. Erwin, Robert J. C. McLean, Gary M. Aron(2011) 'Bacteriophage ecology in Escherichia coli and Pseudomonas aeruginosa mixed-biofilm communities,' *Applied and Environmental Microbiology*, 77(3), pp. 821–829.

Khalifa, Leron, Yair Brosh, Daniel Gelman, Shunit Coppenhagen-Glazer, Shaul Beyth, Ronit Poradosu-Cohen, Yok-Ai Que, Nurit Beyth, and Ronen Hazan. (2015) 'Targeting Enterococcus faecalis biofilms with phage therapy,' *Applied and Environmental Microbiology*, 81(8), pp. 2696–2705.

Kiro, R., Shitrit, D. and Qimron, U. (2014) 'Efficient engineering of a bacteriophage genome using the type IE CRISPR-Cas system,' *RNA Biology*, 11(1), pp. 42–44.

Klare, Ingo, Carola Konstabel, Dietlinde Badstübner, Guido Werner, and Wolfgang Witte(2003) 'Occurrence and spread of antibiotic resistances in Enterococcus faecium,' *International Journal of Food Microbiology*, 88(2–3), pp. 269–290.

Knezevic, P., D. Obreht, S. Curcin, M. Petrusic, V. Aleksic, R. Kostanjsek, and O. Petrovic (2011) 'Phages of Pseudomonas aeruginosa: response to environmental factors and *in vitro* ability to inhibit bacterial growth and biofilm formation,' *Journal of Applied Microbiology*, 111(1), pp. 245–254.

Kortright, Kaitlyn E., Benjamin K. Chan, Jonathan L. Koff, and Paul E. Turner (2019) 'Phage therapy: a renewed approach to combat antibiotic-resistant bacteria,' *Cell Host & Microbe*, 25(2), pp. 219–232.

Kumar, Manoj, Devojit Kumar Sarma, Swasti Shubham, Manoj Kumawat, Vinod Verma, Praveen Balabaskaran Nina, Devraj Jp, Santosh Kumar, Birbal Singh, and Rajnarayan R. Tiwari(2021) 'Futuristic non-antibiotic therapies to combat antibiotic resistance: A review,' *Frontiers in Microbiology*, p. 16.

Kyriakidis, Ioannis, Eleni Vasileiou, Zoi Dorothea Pana, and Athanasios Tragiannidis. (2021) 'Acinetobacter baumannii antibiotic resistance mechanisms,' *Pathogens*, 10(3), p. 373.

Lambert, P. (2002) 'Mechanisms of antibiotic resistance in Pseudomonas aeruginosa,' *Journal of the Royal Society of Medicine*, 95(Suppl 41), p. 22.

Lee, A. S. Hermínia de Lencastre, Javier Garau, Jan Kluytmans, Surbhi Malhotra-Kumar, Andreas Peschel & Stephan Harbarth.(2018) 'Methicillin-resistant Staphylococcus aureus,' *Nature Reviews Disease Primers*, 4(1), pp. 1–23.

Lee, Chang-Ro, Jung Hun Lee, Moonhee Park, Kwang Seung Park, Il Kwon Bae, Young Bae Kim, Chang-Jun Cha, Byeong Chul Jeong, and Sang Hee Lee (2017) 'Biology of Acinetobacter baumannii: pathogenesis, antibiotic resistance mechanisms, and prospective treatment options,' *Frontiers in Cellular and Infection Microbiology*, p. 55.

Lenneman, Bryan R, Jonas Fernbach, Martin J Loessner, Timothy K Lu, and Samuel Kilcher.(2021) 'Enhancing phage therapy through synthetic biology and genome engineering,' *Current Opinion in Biotechnology*, 68, pp. 151–159.

Loc-Carrillo, C. and Abedon, S. T. (2011) 'Pros and cons of phage therapy,' *Bacteriophage*, 1(2), pp. 111–114.

Lood, Rolf, Benjamin Y. Winer, Adam J. Pelzek, Roberto Diez-Martinez, Mya Thandar, Chad W. Euler, Raymond Schuch, and Vincent A. Fischetti (2015) 'Novel phage lysin capable of killing the multidrug-resistant gram-negative bacterium Acinetobacter baumannii in a mouse bacteremia model,' *Antimicrobial Agents and Chemotherapy*, 59(4), pp. 1983–1991.

Lowy, F. D. (2003) 'Antimicrobial resistance: the example of Staphylococcus aureus,' *The Journal of Clinical Investigation*, 111(9), pp. 1265–1273.

Marinelli, Laura J., Mariana Piuri, Zuzana Swigoňová, Amrita Balachandran, Lauren M. Oldfield, Julia C. van Kessel, and Graham F. Hatfull. (2008) 'BRED: a simple and powerful tool for constructing mutant and recombinant bacteriophage genomes,' *PLoS One*, 3(12), p. e3957.

Martel, B. and Moineau, S. (2014) 'CRISPR-Cas: an efficient tool for genome engineering of virulent bacteriophages,' *Nucleic Acids Research*, 42(14), pp. 9504–9513.

Mayo-Muñoz, David, Fei He, Jacob Jørgensen, Poul Madsen, Yuvaraj Bhoobalan-Chitty, and Xu Peng. (2018) 'Anti-CRISPR-based and CRISPR-based genome editing of Sulfolobus islandicus rod-shaped virus 2,' *Viruses*, 10(12), p. 695.

Moelling, K., Broecker, F. and Willy, C. (2018) 'A wake-up call: we need phage therapy now,' *Viruses*, 10(12), p. 688.

Mulani, Mansura S., Ekta E. Kamble, Shital N. Kumkar, Madhumita S. Tawre, and Karishma R. Pardesi. (2019) 'Emerging strategies to combat ESKAPE pathogens in the era of antimicrobial resistance: a review,' *Frontiers in Microbiology*, 10, p. 539.

Nilsson, A. S. (2019) 'Pharmacological limitations of phage therapy,' *Upsala Journal of Medical Sciences*, 124(4), pp. 218–227.

Nir-Paz, R. Daniel Gelman, Ayman Khouri4, Brittany M Sisson, Joseph Fackler, Sivan Alkalay-Oren, Leron Khalifa, Amit Rimon, Ortal Yerushalmy, Reem Bader, Sharon Amit, Shunit Coppenhagen-Glazer, Matthew Henry, Javier Quinones, Francisco Malagon, Biswajit Biswas, Allon E Moses, Greg Merril, Robert T Schooley, Michael J Brownstein, Yoram A Weil, Ronen Hazan. (2019) 'Successful treatment of antibiotic-resistant, poly-microbial bone infection with bacteriophages and antibiotics combination,' *Clinical Infectious Diseases*, 69(11), pp. 2015–2018.

Patil, A., Banerji, R., Kanojiya, P. and Saroj, S. D. (2021) 'Foodborne ESKAPE biofilms and antimicrobial resistance: lessons learned from clinical isolates,' *Pathogens and Global Health*, 115(6), pp. 339–356.

Patil, Amrita, Rajashri Banerji, Poonam Kanojiya, Santosh Koratkar, and Sunil Saroj. (2021) 'Bacteriophages for ESKAPE: Role in pathogenicity and measures of control,' *Expert Review of Anti-Infective Therapy*, 19(7), pp. 845–865.

Paul, K., Merabishvili, M., Hazan, R., Christner, M., Herden, U., Gelman, D., Khalifa, L., Yerushalmy, O., Coppenhagen-Glazer, S., Harbauer, T., Schulz-Jürgensen, S., Rohde, H., Fischer, L., Aslam, S., Rohde, C., Nir-Paz, R., Pirnay, J.-P., Singer, D., & Muntau, A. C. (2021) 'Bacteriophage Rescue Therapy of a Vancomycin-Resistant Enterococcus faecium Infection in a One-Year-Old Child following a Third Liver Transplantation,' *Viruses*, 13(9), p. 1785.

Payaslian, F., Gradaschi, V. and Piuri, M. (2021) 'Genetic manipulation of phages for therapy using BRED,' *Current Opinion in Biotechnology*, 68, pp. 8–14.

Peleg, A. Y., Seifert, H. and Paterson, D. L. (2008) 'Acinetobacter baumannii: emergence of a successful pathogen,' *Clinical Microbiology Reviews*, 21(3), pp. 538–582.

Pines, Gur, Emily F. Freed, James D. Winkler, and Ryan T. Gill. (2015) 'Bacterial recombineering: genome engineering via phage-based homologous recombination,' *ACS Synthetic Biology*, 4(11), pp. 1176–1185.

Pires, Diana P., Sara Cleto, Sanna Sillankorva, Joana Azeredo, and Timothy K. Lu. (2016) 'Genetically engineered phages: a review of advances over the last decade,' *Microbiology and Molecular Biology Reviews*, 80(3), pp. 523–543.

Rice, L. B. (2010) 'Progress and challenges in implementing the research on ESKAPE pathogens,' *Infection Control & Hospital Epidemiology*, 31(S1), pp. S7–S10.

Rita Costa, A. Catarina Milho, Joana Azeredo, Diana Priscila Pires. (2018) 'Synthetic biology to engineer bacteriophage genomes,' in *Bacteriophage Therapy*. Springer, pp. 285–300.

Schooley, R. T., Biswas, B., Gill, J. J., Hernandez-Morales, A., Lancaster, J., Lessor, L., Barr, J. J., Reed, S. L., Rohwer, F., Benler, S., Segall, A. M., Taplitz, R., Smith, D. M., Kerr, K., Kumaraswamy, M., Nizet, V., Lin, L., McCauley, M. D., Strathdee, S. A., Hamilton, T. (2017) 'Development and use of personalized bacteriophage-based therapeutic cocktails to treat a patient with a disseminated resistant Acinetobacter baumannii infection,' *Antimicrobial Agents and Chemotherapy*, 61(10), pp. e00954-17.

Shin, J., Jardine, P. and Noireaux, V. (2012) 'Genome replication, synthesis, and assembly of the bacteriophage T7 in a single cell-free reaction,' *ACS Synthetic Biology*, 1(9), pp. 408–413.

Shrivastava, S. R., Shrivastava, P. S. and Ramasamy, J. (2018) 'World health organization releases global priority list of antibiotic-resistant bacteria to guide research, discovery, and development of new antibiotics,'*Journal of Medical Society*, 32(1), p. 76.

Silva, Carina, Sara Sá, Carla Guedes, Carla Oliveira, Cláudio Lima, Marco Oliveira, João Mendes, Gonçalo Novais, Pilar Baylina, and Ruben Fernandes. (2021) 'The History and Applications of Phage Therapy in Pseudomonas aeruginosa,' *Microbiology Research*, 13(1), pp. 14–37.

Stern, A. and Sorek, R. (2011) 'The phage-host arms race: shaping the evolution of microbes,' *Bioessays*, 33(1), pp. 43–51.

Sulakvelidze, A., Alavidze, Z. and Morris Jr, J. G. (2001) 'Bacteriophage therapy,' *Antimicrobial Agents and Chemotherapy*, 45(3), pp. 649–659.

Sulis, G., Sayood, S., Katukoori, S., Bollam, N., George, I., Yaeger, L. H., Chavez, M. A., Tetteh, E., Yarrabelli, S., Pulcini, C., Harbarth, S., Mertz, D., Sharland, M., Moja, L., Huttner, B., & Gandra, S. (2022) 'Exposure to WHO AWaRe antibiotics and isolation of multi-drug resistant bacteria: a systematic review and meta-analysis,' *Clinical Microbiology and Infection*.

Tabassum, Rabia, Muafia Shafique, Komal Amer Khawaja, Iqbal Ahmed Alvi, Yasir Rehman, Cody S. Sheik, Zaigham Abbas, and Shafiq ur Rehman(2018) 'Complete genome analysis of a Siphoviridae phage TSK1 showing biofilm removal potential against Klebsiella pneumoniae,'*Scientific Reports*, 8(1), pp. 1–11.

Taha, Omar A., Phillippa L. Connerton, Ian F. Connerton, and Ayman El-Shibiny(2018) 'Bacteriophage ZCKP1: a potential treatment for Klebsiella pneumoniae isolated from diabetic foot patients,' *Frontiers in Microbiology*, p. 2127.

Thwaites, Guy E, Jonathan D Edgeworth, Effrossyni Gkrania-Klotsas, Andrew Kirby, Robert Tilley, M Estée Török, Sarah Walker, Heiman FL Wertheim, Peter Wilson, and Martin J Llewelyn. (2011) 'Clinical management of Staphylococcus aureus bacteraemia,' *The Lancet Infectious Diseases*, 11(3), pp. 208–222.

Tinoco, Justine Monnerat, Bettina Buttaro, Hongming Zhang, Nadia Liss, Luciana Sassone, and Roy Stevens. (2016) 'Effect of a genetically engineered bacteriophage on Enterococcus faecalis biofilms,' *Archives of Oral Biology*, 71, pp. 80–86.

Tümmler, B. (2019) 'Emerging therapies against infections with Pseudomonas aeruginosa,' *F1000Research*, 8.

Twort, F. W. (1961) 'An investigation on the nature of ultra-microscopic viruses,' *Acta Kravsi*.

van Hal, S. J., Willems, R. J. L., Gouliouris, T., Ballard, S. A., Coque, T. M., Hammerum, A. M., Hegstad, K., Westh, H. T., Howden, B. P., Malhotra-Kumar, S., Werner, G., Yanagihara, K., Earl, A. M., Raven, K. E., Corander, J., & Bowden, R.(2021) 'The global dissemination of hospital clones of Enterococcus faecium,'*Genome Medicine*, 13(1), pp. 1–12.

Victor L Yu, Dennis S Hansen, Wen Chien Ko, Asia Sagnimeni, Keith P Klugman, Anne von Gottberg, Herman Goossens, Marilyn M Wagener, Vicente J Benedi, International Klebseilla Study Group.(2007) 'Virulence characteristics of Klebsiella and clinical manifestations of K. pneumoniae bloodstream infections,' *Emerging Infectious Diseases*, 13(7), p. 986.

Wright, A. C. H. Hawkins, E. E. Anggård, D. R. Harper. (2009) 'A controlled clinical trial of a therapeutic bacteriophage preparation in chronic otitis due to antibiotic-resistant Pseudomonas aeruginosa; a preliminary report of efficacy,' *Clinical Otolaryngology*, 34(4), pp. 349–357.

## Chapter 5

# Pathogenesis of Opportunistic Infections

## Salini Krishnarao Kandhalu* and K. V. Murali Mohan
Department of Pathology,
Maharajah Institute of Medical Sciences,
Nellimarla, Vizianagaram Andhra Pradesh, India

### Abstract

Opportunistic infections (OIs) are caused by a non-pathogenic microorganism in an immunocompromised individual. OIs causing organisms are bacteria, viruses, fungi, and parasites which are commonly present in the environment and also in immunocompetent individuals. These organisms become pathogenic and infectious when there is an imbalance between host immunity and virulence of the pathogen. Typically, the balance is maintained by our immune system which can be natural or acquired immunity. In human, natural immunity is inborn and pre-programmed at the time of birth, whereas the adaptive is stimulated naturally or by artificial means to build immunity and do the defense mechanism. The immunity is lost or reduced under certain circumstances includes genetic mutations, chromosomal abnormality, autoimmune destruction of immune cells, environmental predisposition damage to immune cells, specific infections which have tropism for the immune cells and destroy them, major trauma and injuries, nutritional deficiency and therapy for cancers with immunosuppressants. There are a few well-known conditions like Diabetes Mellitus, HIV, organ or bone marrow transplantation, covid-19 are at most risk for this OIs. Notably, patients who need to be started on prophylactic drugs to prevent OIs as the defense mechanism in the immune system is reduced and cause the

---

* Corresponding Author's Email: shalinigkf@gmail.com.

In: Interdisciplinary Approaches on Opportunistic Infections ...
Editors: Jayapradha Ramakrishnan and Ganesh Babu Malli Mohan
ISBN: 978-1-68507-984-0
© 2022 Nova Science Publishers, Inc.

non-pathogenic organism to grow in large number. Immunity in a host can be maintained by means of good control of infection with appropriate therapy for the above diseases. The conclusion is that immunity is the main weapon for an individual to protect against OIs as well the other infections which would help to lead a healthy normal life.

**Keywords:** opportunistic infections, immunity, HIV vs ART, AIDS, uncontrolled diabetes, post-transplant infection, immunodeficiency causing infection

## 1. Introduction

Opportunistic infections (OIs) are infections triggered by non-pathogenic microorganisms, which become pathogenic when the immune system is weakened due to an unrelated disease or other means. OIs can be caused by Viruses, Bacteria, Fungi, and Parasites. These OIs occurs when there is a loss of balance between the host immunity (decrease) and the virulence of the organism (increased). The major cause of the loss of host immunity is by the loss of immune fighting cells. This decrease in defense leads to the relaxation of microorganisms at the checkpoint in cell proliferation causing overgrowth (Cooper, 2009). They become a surplus in the body and escape the counteraction from our immune system. Infections that are generally of lower virulence within a healthy host, whereas the infection in weakened immune system cause more severe and frequent diseases, especially in immunosuppressed individuals and they tend to be more resistant to conventional therapies used for the general population.

Infections are labeled as opportunistic infections only when the organism has certain characteristic features, such as (Shanson, 1989):

1. Low pathogenicity
2. Causing serious infections on impairment of host defense mechanisms
3. Behaving as a conventional pathogen and causes atypical clinical presentation

## 2. Predisposing Factor for Opportunistic Infections

One of the important causes of an opportunistic infection is destructive treatments for malignant diseases. Chemotherapy approaches and other accomplishments of the last decades in medical science confer longer survival with a disease were previously considered untreatable (Riccardi et al., 2019a). As every treatment is obtained at a cost and our immunity under risk which provide a space for low virulent pathogens to grow and become virulent to cause OIs. This remains a major cause of therapy-associated morbidity and mortality. Neutropenia (decreased white blood cells) presents the most significant risk factor for OIs, which is directly associated with its duration and severity. Mild neutropenia gives rise to a bacterial infection and as the white cell count decreases the possibility of infection with viruses, parasite, and fungus (Dean, 2021) increases rapidly and can also get resistant to routine management.

The most common diseases that cause weakening of the immune system and trigger the OIs are:

1. HIV
2. Diabetes Mellitus
3. Malignancy /cancer
4. Organ or bone marrow transplant
5. COVID-19.

We will discuss these particular diseases and the common opportunistic infections seen in people who have them throughout this chapter.

## 3. Routes of Transmission of Opportunistic Infections

Microorganisms have the propensity to spread via various routes. The most important one is via aerosol which being the most common while others like body fluids, contaminated food, water, direct inoculation, person to person, etc. (Tellier et al., 2019). Hospital: Co-workers, doctors, patients, relatives, instruments, and other equipment in the hospital also take part in transmitting the infection.

Before going into the pathogenesis of opportunistic infections let us learn about our immune system and its function briefly.

Immunity is the defense mechanism of a living being (humans as well as other species).

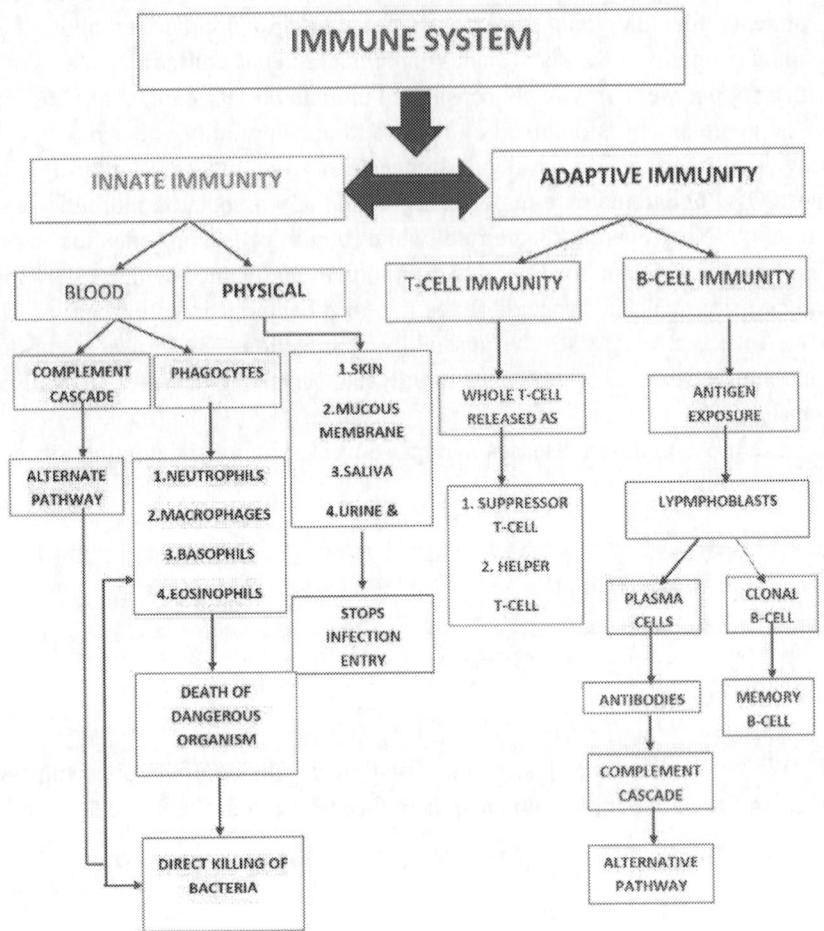

**Figure 1.** Schematic representation of a fundamentals of the immune system.

## 4. Fundamentals of the Immune System

### 4.1. Innate Immunity

Innate immunity refers to a non-specific initial defense mechanism triggered upon pathogenic recognition. It is also called "IN BORN" or "NATIVE"

Immunity and it is similar in all the individuals of the same species and it is pre-programmed (Sun et al., 2020). Innate immunity makes up a set of disease resistance mechanisms, which is not specific to any particular disease-causing organism, but recognizes a class of molecules common to most frequently encountered infection caused by the microorganism. This immunity gives immediate protection that it has no time lag, doesn't need a memory to be reminded on exposure to the infection-causing organism. It does not have any antigen specificity.

A. Barriers of Innate Immunity
1. *Physical Barriers*: includes, skin, hair, cilia, mucous membrane, mucosal secretions, saliva, digestive enzymes, and acid secretion in the stomach.
2. *Blood Born Barriers*
   a. Cellular Examples: Phagocytes (Neutrophils, basophils, eosinophils, dendritic cells, and macrophages) which are primary defense mechanism of the host cell.
   b. Humoral Examples: complements, chemokines, interleukins, leukotrienes, interferons, and so on.

## 4.2. Adaptive Immunity or Acquired Immunity

Acquired immune response is also known as "adaptive" because the host's body prepares the immune system to be proactive and to fight against future challenging pathogens. This acquired immunity is a subsystem of immunity which is made up of specific systemic cells and processes that remove infection causing organism/pathogens or inhibit their growth. In vertebrates, an adaptive immunity comprises one among the two chief immune strategies. This system includes both humoral immunity and cell-mediated immunity components which help in destroying the entering pathogens. Contrasting the innate immune system which non-specific and pre-programmed to react to broad categories of common pathogen, the adaptive immune system is highly specific to certain pathogens the body encountered (Smith et al., 2019).

The white blood cells bring the adaptive immune responses are known as lymphocytes - T cells and B cells they carry out the main defense activity against the offending pathogen. 1) cell-mediated immune response, and 2) antibody response respectively. T cells are activated to function as helper (CD4), cytotoxic (CD8), and suppressor cells. In antibody response B-cell gets activated and antibodies are secreted which are known as immunoglobulins (Ig). These antibodies (Ig) travel into the bloodstream and bind to the foreign agents termed antigen, causing them to inactivate and prevent the antigen binding to the host (B Cells and Antibodies - Molecular Biology of the Cell - NCBI Bookshelf, n.d.).

Adaptive immunity has 2 types: 1) *Active* and 2) *Passive*. These 2 types can be acquired naturally or artificially. A common type of adaptive immunity is Active Immunity, and it develops in response to an infection/vaccine.

### *4.2.1. Natural – By Infection*

Upon exposure to an infection by an organism or pathogen, naturally our body immune system gets activated. T cell and B cell recognize these pathogens as invaders and start the defense mechanism and eliminate the offending organism or pathogen. As our immune system develops a memory cell on exposure to the pathogens, the same memory cells will activate by the immune cells much faster than the previous response with very less stimulus from the offending pathogen (Nicholson, 2016). Thus, the immunological memory prevents a host from getting repeated and severe infections from the same organism.

### *4.2.2 Artificial – Vaccination*

Artificial active immunity has a similar action as that of natural immunity, but these immune cells are activated by injecting a small amount of infection causing organism. There might be mild infectivity symptoms, but does not cause the infection.

Adaptive immunity can provide temporary and long-term protection. Most of the natural immunity are lifelong but the artificial one depends on the host immune response and the type of vaccine given (live, live attenuated, killed). For example, someone who recovers from measles and chicken pox is now protected of their lifetime. However, vaccination given for infection does not provide lifetime protection and requires booster doses to maintain an immune fighting cell amounts in the body. Antibodies are a crucial part of the adaptive immune system, thus immunity or the protection depends upon the number of antibodies produced inside the host Dose-dependent. This process of adaptive immunity is the root of vaccination (The Adaptive Immune System - Molecular Biology of the Cell - NCBI Bookshelf, n.d.).

Passive immunity is developed in the host is developed after receiving the preformed antibodies or the immunoglobulins. As our acquired immunity is a dose dependent this form of passive immunity is temporary which is not produced by the host and instead received from other sources. The immune cells are not activated and there is no immunological memory for future infection in passive immunity. The source of an immunity can be natural or artificial (Marcotte & Hammarström, 2015).

### 4.2.2.1. Natural – By Maternal Antibodies

Newborn receives preformed antibodies from a mother which usually transfer during pregnancy through a placenta or exclusively through mothers' breast milk after birth, here comes the importance of breastfeeding and the protection received by the infant completely until 6 months of age. This protection is maximum in infants who are exclusively breastfeed for 6 months (Niewiesk, 2014).

### 4.2.2.2. Artificial – By Ig Treatments

An Ig are pooled antibodies obtained from previous infected hosts; these immunoglobulins are usually employed to treat patients at risk for infections. Eg: After snakebite, newborns of Hepatitis positive mothers. These antibodies are developed in a research lab or collected from other people or animals.

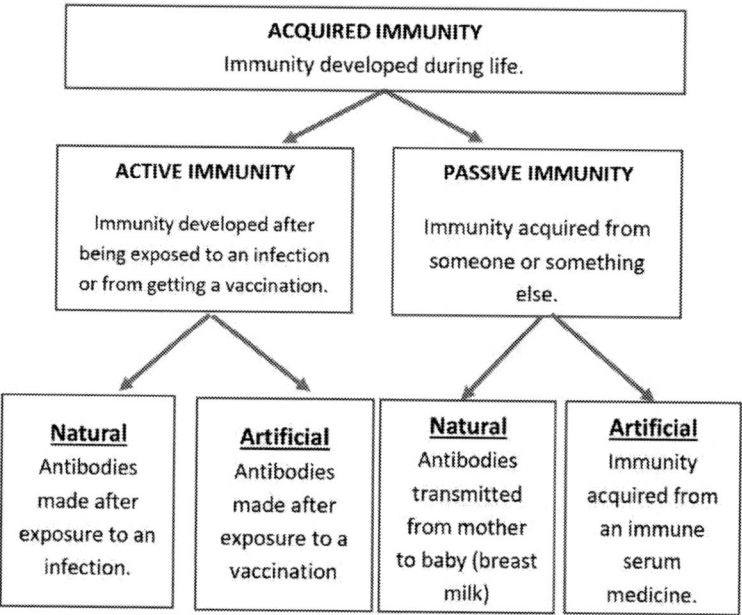

**Figure 2.** Acquired immunity.

**Table 1.** Differences in innate and adaptive immune response

|  | Innate Immune Response | Adaptive Immune Response |
| --- | --- | --- |
| Takes Effect | Instantly | Slow and overtime |
| Response Type | Non-specific | Specific |
| Types | External defense<br>Internal defense | Active immunity (natural and artificial)<br>Passive immunity (natural and artificial) |
| Also Known as | Natural immunity<br>Inborn immunity | Acquired immunity |
| Length of Efficacy | Lifelong | Short-term, long-term, lifelong |

## 5. Causes for the Reduced Host Immunity

*A naturally impaired immune system:*

- Physiological: A very young age and old age (i.e. extremes of ages) which could be transient (pregnancy, illness) or long term.
- Genetic: Immunodeficiency syndrome (i.e.) defect and deletion of genes causing breakage in the chromosomes, enzyme deficiency, altered metabolism, loss of normal cell regulation; sporadic-acquired mutation, Genomic instability, epigenetic variation, etc.
- Environmental: Radiation, chemical, toxins causing damage to the immune system.
- Malnutrition: Deficiency in diet or malabsorption.

*An impaired immune system:*

- Disease related - Immune cell destruction
  - An example is T-cell/ CD4 helper loss in cases of HIV infection.
- Treatment related- Immunosuppressant use
  - Examples:
    - Autoimmune disease- immunosuppressor.
    - Cancer (chemotherapy, radiotherapy).
    - Transplant organ or bone marrow related therapy.
    - Post-op low immunity.
    - Skin disease treatment with steroids.
    - Anti-Inflammatory drugs.

## Pathogenesis of Opportunistic Infections

- Prolonged antibiotic therapy.
- Prolonged Proton pump inhibitor use(antacids)
- Metabolic
  - Examples:
    - Diabetes
    - Anemia (Low Hemoglobin).
    - Cushing's syndrome excess natural steroid).
    - Malnutrition.

A few conditions and diseases which are at most risk of this OI is Diabetes mellitus type 1 & 2, HIV infection, covid -19, immunodeficiency diseases, malnutrition, prolonged immunosuppressants, post-organ and stem cell transplant.

**Table 2.** Immune status alteration and the list of causative agents with the treatment options

| Causative agent | Immune status | Organism in particular | Treatment |
|---|---|---|---|
| Bacterial | Mild dysfunction | Mycobacterium Tuberculosis, Clostridium difficle, Pseudomonas, Legionella, Staphylococcus aureus, Streptococcus, Salmonella. | Broad spectrum antibiotics. |
| Virus | Moderate dysfunction | Herpes Simplex, Cytomegalovirus, Human herpes virus 8, JC virus, HIV. | Antiviral, Boosting the immune system. |
| Fungus | Severe dysfunction | Aspergillus, Coccoidimitis, Histoplasmosis, Pneumocystis Carni pneumonia, Candida, Mucormycosis. | Antifungal, Boosting the immune system. |
| Parasite | Severe dysfunction | Cryptosporidium, Toxoplasma | Anti-helminths, Removing the offending agent, Boosting the immune system. |

## 5.1. Diabetes Mellitus (DM)

DM is a clinical syndrome connected with a deficiency in the secretion of insulin or reduced action in the peripheral tissues. It is one of the largest evolving threats to health in the 21$^{st}$ century. According to the current data, it is estimated that more than 380 million people with DM in 2025 (Atkins & Zimmet, 2010) along with the classical and common complications of the disease, DM has been associated with the decreased response of T cells, neutrophil function (white blood cell), and disorders of humoral immunity (Geerlings & Hoepelman, 1999; Muller et al., 2005; Peleg et al., 2007). Consequently, DM rises the susceptibility of infections to the most common ones, as well as always affect only people with DM (e.g., Rhino-orbito-cerebral Mucormycosis) (Peleg et al., 2007) which potentially increases the disability and death.

The main pathogenic mechanisms for causing reduced immunity and allowing the normal commensals to cause opportunistic infection are:

1. Hyperglycemia increasing the virulence of few pathogens by providing an ambient environment to grow and as well as reducing the Interleukins production in response to infection.
2. Reduced chemotaxis and phagocytosis, neutrophils immobilization, glycosuria, Gastrointestinal and Genitourinary dysmotility, Micro- and macro-angiopathies, neuropathy, decrease in the antibacterial activity of urine, and a greater number of medical interventions in these patients like using arterial lines, urinary catheters, frequent insulin injection, etc.

Additionally, in DM metabolic complications like hypoglycemia, ketoacidosis, and coma are increased in the presence of an OI. Infections affect organs and systems such as foot infections, malignant external otitis, rhino-orbito-cerebral Mucormycosis, and gangrenous cholecystitis. Furthermore, to the increased morbidity, infectious processes may be the initial manifestation of DM or the precipitating factors for hitches inherent to the disease, such as diabetic ketoacidosis and hypoglycemia.

*Important note:* The recommendation of compulsory immunization with anti-pneumococcal vaccine is essential because this vaccine could reduce major respiratory infections and the number of deaths related to respiratory tract disease. Regular vaccination can also reduce the burden of medical expenses needed for the number and length of hospitalization.

*The common OIs in diabetes patients are:*

### 5.1.1. Malignant Otitis External

External otitis as the name suggests is an infection of the external ear. It is a serious infection but not cancer or tumor (malignant). As the infection is severe and spreads very rapidly and is associated with high morbidity and mortality it is termed as malignant. It is an invasive disease that can spread to nearby structures and also to the central nervous system affecting the base of brain (skull) and cranial nerves (Joshi et al., 1999; Magliocca et al., 2018). The infection can involve the facial bones causing osteomyelitis. This infection commonly affects elderly patients and the causative agent is *Pseudomonas aeruginosa* (Carfrae & Kesser, 2008; Magliocca et al., 2018; Rubin & Yu, 1988).

   a. *Clinical features:* Patients usually present with severe excruciating pain, which is very severe at night and they don't tend to respond to topical medication or home treatment. Discharge from ear, hearing loss (Carfrae & Kesser, 2008) cranial nerve palsies - especially facial nerve involvement is noted in at least 50% of patients (Magliocca et al., 2018).
   b. *Diagnosis*: The best diagnostic method of investigation is Magnetic resonance imaging (Magliocca et al., 2018) Malignant otitis externa requires immediate intervention with medical and or surgical management to prevent complications.
   c. *Treatment:* Treatment options depend upon the site and severity of the infection. A mild infection responds well and subsides with medical management with DM control. An invasive infection requires surgical exploration followed by aggressive medical therapy along with strict diabetes control and other supportive measures.

### 5.1.2. Rhinoorbitocerebral Mucormycosis

Mucormycosis is a lethal opportunistic infection caused by filamentous fungi of family (mucoracea). It is also a rare opportunistic and invasive infection caused by Zygomycetes (Artal et al., 2010; Giuliani et al., 2010). The most common association with human infections is specific genus and they are a *Rhizopus*, followed by *Mucor* and *Cunninghamella* (Severo et al., 2010). Classically, major risk factors for Mucormycosis coupled with immuno-suppressive conditions such as uncontrolled diabetes mellitus (DM), neutropenia, immunosuppressive therapy like chemotherapy and corticosteroid (Cornely et al., 2019).

1. *Routes of acquiring infection*
   Inhalation of spores is the main route of infection as this fungus is present ubiquitously in the decaying organic matter occurring in the soil. It can cause infection of the lungs, paranasal sinuses, orbit, gastrointestinal tract, and the skin. The commonest affected organ is lungs followed by paranasal sinuses. However, soft tissue and cutaneous invasion occurs after skin disruption caused by traumatic injuries, surgery, or burns (Cornely et al., 2019).
2. *Diagnosis*
   Diagnosis of mucormycosis comprises clinical, microscopic imaging modalities alongside histopathology, cultures, and molecular techniques (Skiada et al., 2020).
3. *Mechanism*
   This infection occurs in approximately 50% of the cases in patients with DM due to the huge amount of glucose availability for pathogen which provides a favorable environment for the mucor to grow. The reduction in serum inhibitory activity against the *Rhizopus* under lower pH, and the induced expression of few host receptors mediates the invasion and damage to epithelial cells by *Rhizopus* (Calvet & Yoshikawa, 2001; Liu et al., 2010).
4. *Clinical features*
   The mucormycosis can be acute and chronic.
   The classical triad of mucormycosis is paranasal sinusitis, ophthalmoplegia (muscular defect) with blindness, and unilateral proptosis with cellulitis (Artal et al., 2010). Patients clinically present with headache, swelling, and redness of eyes associated with facial pain, eye pain, decreased vision, double vision, reduced smell or nasal blockage and also black discharge from the nose. Necrotic wound of the palate of the nasal mucosa called the eschar. Black necrotic eschar in the nasal cornets is a characteristic sign (Casqueiro et al., 2012; Nagasawa et al., 2010). Mucormycosis has a tendency for angioinvasion, which means spreading through blood vessels and thus can cause thrombosis (blockage of the blood vessels and reduce the blood flow) and interfere with cell survival and lead to cell death. This leads to formation of black necrotic eschar and thus mucormycosis is called black fungus.

5. *Treatment*
Mild infections are treated medically with systemic antifungals as early as possible. Moderate to severe infection require endoscopic sinus debridement along with antifungals. Stopping immunosuppressive drugs at the earliest and change to available and sensitive alternatives. Also, patients are started on prophylactic and supportive medication to prevent other infections.

## 5.2. COVID-19-Associated Opportunistic Infections

The current pandemic with COVID-19 has caused the reduction in host immunity and is the major cause for OI. It affects people at extremes of age and people with other comorbidities.

The route of spread is via aerosol and droplet thus causing it an easy mode of spread of an infection. The upper respiratory tract and lungs are a commonly affected parts of the host as the virus are more attracted to the receptors in the lungs. An important concern is to be provided especially to patients with underlying diseases like diabetes, immunodeficiency diseases, pregnancy, extremes of age, and in patients who are on immunosuppressive therapy for various disorders (Clementi et al., 2021). COVID-19 has been associated with a wide range of OI with bacteria, virus, and fungi. Steroids, which is a lifesaving treatment for severe and critically ill COVID-19 patients but might be the trigger for fungal infections. These steroids and immunosuppressive therapy control the dysregulated immune response following coronavirus infection, as in case of cytokine storm syndrome where our bodily defense response itself causing self-destruction and it acts like a double-edged sword thus this has to be used wisely.

These opportunistic infections are specifically detected in uncontrolled Diabetic mellitus patients and people on a prolonged use of steroids which may be used as per recommendation or inappropriately. As the upper airway and lungs are affected the adequate oxygen carrying capacity is reduced leading to hypoxia and it is the mandatory requirement of oxygen supplementation through an oxygen mask, re-breathable mask, CPAP, and finally, the last resort being the mechanical ventilators which does the artificial effort of breathing (O'Driscoll et al., 2008). These are only supportive measures. The mechanical ventilators are known to be the breeding grounds and the entry point for these deadly pathogens in critically ill patients with COVID-19 infection.

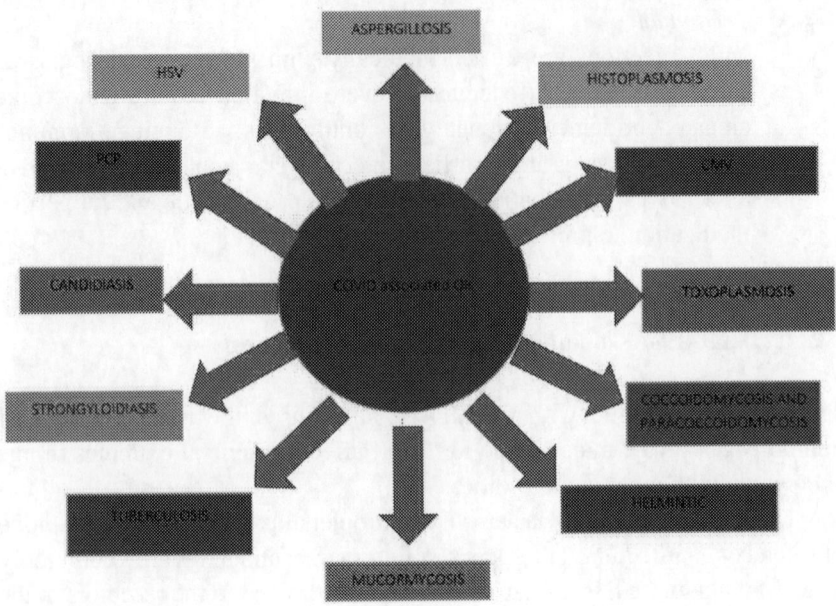

Figure 3. Complications of COVID-19 infection.

The correct medicine for covid-19 is under research. Most of the viruses are volatile that they tend to change its property by means of mutation and thus developing vaccines or finding the exact medication is difficult. The antiviral can reduce the viral load but cannot eradicate the complete infection. Steroids can control the hyperresponsiveness of our body to the virus and thus prevents the cytokine storm syndrome which by itself is fatal.

Among the opportunistic infections, fungal infections account for a most case reports in COVID-19 patients. The common fungal infections are *Aspergillosis* and *Mucormycosis*. Thus, patients suspected for moderate severity or with risk factors like Diabetes, old age, patients on immunosuppressants should have frequent close monitoring and also should be started on prophylactic antifungals/ antivirals. Approximately threefold higher in an individual's mortality rates with diabetes compared to the common mortality of COVID-19 (O'Driscoll et al., 2008). The most important way of prevention is getting vaccination as per the medical experts' advice.

Preventive measures for COVID-19:

1. Wearing face mask.
2. Maintaining social distance.

3. Frequent hand washing with soaps and water or alcohol-based solutions.
4. Avoid getting out of the house or traveling.
5. Healthy and nutritional diet.
6. Use of prophylaxis in high-risk individuals.
7. Vaccination as per government and medical expert advice.
8. Immediate medical attention if any symptoms like fever, sore throat, cough with breathing difficulty.
9. Not to believe unnecessary false information's from the common people.
10. Isolation and follow quarantine rules if detected positive.

## 5.3. Human Immunodeficiency Virus (HIV)

Human Immunodeficiency Virus by name itself is self-explanatory that this virus causes decreased immunity, especially cellular immunity which we had learnt in detail from the basics of immunity.

As we all know that having HIV/AIDS means weekend immune system. The virus destroys the white blood cells which defend from all kinds of infection. HIV classically reduces the CD4 cells by destruction and decreased production of it in the host. These are the helper cells of our immune system. The reduction in CD4 counts puts host at risk for common infections and opportunistic infections. Among those diagnosed with HIV, approximately half of the patients had been infected by HIV at least 3 years ago (Bacchetti et al., 1988). Also, approximately 1 in 5 required a CD4 T lymphocyte (CD4) cell count which is less than 200 cells/mm3 for a diagnosis to be made. These infections are less common and less severe in healthy people and having HIV/AIDS make these infections difficult to treat. On an average of 7 to 10 years after infection with HIV, these opportunistic infections were the first symptoms with which patients presented and that made physicians suspect acquired immunodeficiency syndrome (AIDS). Until an effective antiretroviral therapy (ART) was developed, patients had survived only a maximum of 2 years after the classical symptoms of AIDS (Bacchetti et al., 1988). The current recommendation for OIs in HIV patients is to start ART therapy. The therapy will increase host immunity as well as beneficial in preventing OIs (*Mandell, Douglas, and Bennett's Principles and P - 9780323482554*, n.d.)

## 5.3.1. Opportunistic Infections in HIV

- *Bacterial*: Mycobacterium tuberculosis, Pneumocystis pneumonia (PCP), Mycobacterium avium complex (MAC) disease affecting the respiratory system.
  *Note:* Tuberculosis is one disease that can affect any organ in the body and it can be primary or secondary (reactivation of dormant tubercular bacilli).
- *Viral*: Cytomegalovirus - affecting retina of the eye and gastro-intestinal tract especially esophagus.
- *Fungal*: Candidiasis (oral and genital-mucocutaneous), Aspergilla – lung, *Mucor*- rhino-orbit, and central nervous system. Cryptococcal meningitis- covering of brain, histoplasmosis- lung
- *Parasitical:* Clostridium difficile - gastrointestinal tract. Toxoplasma - encephalitis of brain, Cryptosporidiosis.

Certain cancers occur with long-standing HIV/AIDS from Human herpes virus 8 causing Kaposi sarcoma – blood vessels. Chronic infection with HIV itself will induce mutation and oncogenesis leading to the development of lymphoma in the central nervous system and it's a hallmark of AIDS.

When certain OIs occur co-infection with tuberculosis and syphilis increases plasma viral load as they gain mutual benefit and causes increased morbidity and mortality by accelerating HIV progression and increasing disease transmission rate. CD4 count plays a major role for acquiring OIs in HIV patients as these are the helper cells of the immune system. When they decline the dormant and the non-pathogenic organism get activated and become pathogenic. Also, the viral load plays a critical role in reducing the CD4 levels, thus all patients with HIV have to be evaluated for the viral load and the CD4 count. This helps in deciding the treatment regimen and the prophylaxis requirement (Powderly, 2010). Regardless of the CD4 count there are some infections that occur at a higher incidence, like tuberculosis, pneumococcal disease and herpes zoster/shingles which classically seen as dermatomal distribution. OIs occurring varies inversely with the CD4 count and the host immune response, however (Dybul et al., 2002) people with HIV/AIDS are also at increased risk to have complications from common diseases such as the flu.

General preventive measures for opportunistic infections in HIV patients are:

1. Antiretroviral medications.
2. Practicing safe sex by using barrier contraception.
3. Washing hands with soap water or alcohol-based solution and more frequently.
4. Avoid uncooked food.

*5.3.1.1. Bacterial Infections*

**5.3.1.1.1. Mycobacterium Tuberculosis (TB) Infection and Disease**
Globally, Tuberculosis (TB) is the foremost cause of both morbidity and mortality among people with HIV. In 2019, an estimated 820,000 people are infected with both HIV and TB and 208,000 deaths (WHO, 2021). Though the overall annual number of worldwide TB patients are relatively unchanged (1.6% average annual rate of decline) while antiretroviral therapy (ART) coverage has expanded.

TB is so dreadful that it is fully manifested within a year for untreated HIV-infected individuals, especially those who are not on antiretroviral therapy(Sonnenberg et al., 2005a). TB bacteria can attack any individual at any CD4 T lymphocyte (CD4) cell count, although the risk of being infected increases with advanced immunodeficiency (Sonnenberg et al., 2005a) (Wood et al., n.d.). Taking the correct regime of ART doesn't bring an individual risk of TB equal to the general population but the risk remains a little higher but lower than the HIV patients who are not on ART.

A. *Routes of Spread*
   - Aerosol/air born- TB bacteria enter host when a host inhales droplets containing Mycobacterium tuberculosis organisms.
   - Inoculation artificially.
   - Close contact with TB infected individual.
   - Local spread within the host.
   - Dissemination via blood to other organs.

B. *Clinical Manifestations of TB Disease*
   - People infected with HIV and having TB disease are usually asymptomatic but have positive sputum cultures (subclinical TB) as the defective host immunity does not react with the

organism. The clinical presentation of TB disease depends upon immunodeficiency in a host. The risk of TB increased with the drop of CD4 count, especially in patients with CD4 counts 200 cells/mm3 immunity drops and leads to immunodeficiency, extrapulmonary (especially lymphadenitis, pleuritis, pericarditis, and meningitis) or disseminated TB frequency increases. Patients usually present with fever, especially evening rise in temperature, night sweats, weight loss, cough and hemoptysis.

C. *Diagnosis of TB*
- Primary
  Initial diagnostic testing for TB disease depends on the symptoms, signs or anatomic site of involvement (e.g., pulmonary, extrapulmonary, genitourinary or central nervous system). Sputum for AFB, gram stain, special stain, culture, chest radiography, cytology, histopathological examination, PCR, and Nucleic acid amplification test.

D. *Latent TB Infection (LTBI)*
- Patients with HIV are evaluated for LTBI at the time of presentation with HIV, nevertheless of their epidemiological risk of TB exposure. The two important and accurate diagnostics tests available for detection of *M. tuberculosis* infection are IGRA (Interferon Gamma Release Assay) and TST (Tuberculin Skin Test) these are the very sensitive test.

E. *Treating TB Disease*
- Advanced immunodeficiency can cause TB to spread rapidly and become a fatal illness if treatment is delayed. Therefore, after the collection of specimens for traditional culture and molecular diagnostic tests, recommended empiric treatment for TB to the patients with symptoms and signs indicative of HIV-related TB. Treatment of TB with HIV is the same as for patients without HIV and should include a primary four-drug regimen which is a combination of isoniazid, rifampicin, ethambutol, and pyrazinamide (Nahid et al., 2016).
- Drug-susceptible TB infected individuals are started with a 2-month (8-week) rigorous phase of 4 drug regimens of - isoniazid, rifampicin, ethambutol, and pyrazinamide (AI). Ethambutol can be stopped after the susceptibility to isoniazid

and rifampicin are confirmed. Thereafter, isoniazid and a rifamycin are utilized in the extension phase of therapy, generally suggested as an additional 4 months (18 weeks) of treatment for uncomplicated TB (AI). DOT supervised by skilled health care workers, and recommended HIV-related TB patients (Sonnenberg et al., 2005b).
- Some patients may require nine months extension of therapy in patients with a positive sputum culture after 2 months of treatment using antitubercular therapy. Cavitary lesions in the lung and military tuberculosis from vascular spread also need prolonged anti-tuberculous therapy. Most extrapulmonary TB can be treated for 6 months, but TB meningitis treated for more than 12 months. Adjunctive corticosteroid therapy is suggested in individuals with HIV to prevent scarring and additional sequel. Early antiretroviral therapy (ART) initiation requires close collaboration between social workers, HIV and TB care centers expertise in the management of ARV regimen selection, close monitoring, potential adjunctive corticosteroid therapy, and support and compliance to services for and by the patients.

F. *Drug-Resistant TB*
- Although a small fraction of TB cases displays drug-resistant TB. When resistance to these medications develops, both first- and second-line alternative combinations of TB medications recommended.

### 5.3.1.1.2. Gastrointestinal Infection

Enteral infections in HIV infected patients are very common, specifically gram-negative organisms. Bacterial enteric infections display 10-times higher than in the general population, but rate decreases with antiretroviral therapy treatment (ART). The risk of enteric infection varies with CD4 T lymphocyte (CD4) count and is highest in AIDS patients (Wood et al., n.d.). Commonest bacteria isolated in HIV-infected adults are *Salmonella, Shigella*, and *Campylobacter*. Also, *Clostridium difficile*-associated infection (CDI) is not uncommon in HIV-infected patients with reduced CD4 counts.

A. *Source and routes of spread*
- MOA, common source enteric infections in HIV-infected patients and consumption of contaminated food or drinking

contaminated water (Wood et al., n.d.). Unprotected intercourse with the HIV-infected person. By direct or indirect feco-oral exposure also increases a risk of infection with *Shigella* and *Campylobacter*. The use of acid suppressers like proton pump inhibitors or antacids increases the risk of bacterial infection.

B. *Clinical Manifestations*
- Self-limited gastroenteritis, severe, and prolonged diarrhea. Associated with fever, blood stool and weight loss.

C. *Diagnosis*
- Routine stool examination, culture, antigen detection test, and special tests like PCR.

D. *Prevention*
- Antimicrobial prophylaxis to prevent bacterial enteric illness.

## 5.3.1.2. Fungal Infections

### 5.3.1.2.1. Mucocutaneous Infection

Mucocutaneous oropharyngeal and esophageal candidiasis are common in patients with HIV infection (Bonacini et al., n.d.; Klein et al., 1984). *Candida albicans* benign the major responsible organism in causing candidiasis and is recognized as an indicator of immune suppression and is frequently observed in patients with CD4 T lymphocyte (CD4) cell counts <200. Vulvovaginal candidiasis not only occurs in HIV infected patients but also occurs in healthy pregnant women (temporary immunosuppression) and uncontrolled diabetes (preferable environment for the organism).

A. *Clinical Manifestations*
- Mucocutaneous candidiasis is characterized by painless, creamy white, plaque-like ulcers occurring on the buccal surface of the oral cavity, palate, oropharyngeal mucosa, or the tongue.

B. *Diagnosis*
- The diagnosis of esophageal candidiasis is often made clinical response to antiretroviral therapy, or visualization of lesions in culture or histopathologic examination.

C. *Prevention*
- In healthy individuals, *Candida* organisms are commensals and normal flora on mucosal surfaces. Prophylaxis to high-risk

cases and timely identification of new patients and treating them with antifungals would prevent complications

### 5.3.1.3. Viral Infections

#### 5.3.1.3.1. Cytomegalovirus Disease

*Cytomegalovirus (CMV)* causes disseminated or localized end-organ disease in HIV people with high immunosuppression, typically in patients with $CD^{4+}$ T lymphocyte cell (CD4) counts <50, who are not getting the treatment or non-compliant to therapy, or not responding to Antiretroviral Therapy (ART) (DeRodriguez et al., 1994; Jabs et al., 2002).

A. *Clinical Manifestations*
- Retinitis is the most common clinical manifestation but can affect other organs also.

B. *Diagnosis*
- The diagnosis of CMV is typically made on the basis of the clinical presentation includes characteristic retinal changes observed during an eye examination and evidence of the virus in tissue by culture or histopathological examination.

C. *Prevention*
- Although, the CMV infection is common in the population, geographic, socioeconomic, racial, and ethnic variances exist in the CMV occurrence (Bate et al., 2010). The primary method for preventing severe CMV disease is diagnosing the early diagnosis of disease and starting the right therapy. Organ failure due to disease is best prevented by giving ART and to keeping the CD4 count >100 cells/mm3.

D. *Treatment*
- CMV retinitis has to be treated with topical application and systemic antivirals with an active contribution of an ophthalmologist well versed the diagnosis and management of retinal disease.

#### 5.3.1.3.2. Varicella-Zoster Viral Diseases

As we already are aware from the above context that Herpes zoster infection in adults does not depend on the CD4 count. ART has been shown to reduce the incidence of herpes zoster in adults with HIV, undoubtedly because of immune restoration, although the risk of herpes zoster remains threefold able to advance in adults with HIV than in the general population.

A. *Clinical Manifestations*
   - Herpes zoster manifests as a group of cutaneous vesicles which are painful with oozing and classical seen in a dermatomal distribution, often associated with constitutional symptoms like fever, myalgia, itching, and weakness (nerve involvement). People with HIV display CD4 counts <200, are at the highest risk of herpes zoster–related complications, with disseminated herpes zoster (Veenstra et al., 1996). The central nervous system (CNS), and involvement of trigeminal, ophthalmic, and facial nerve is some of a temporary favorite area for herpes zoster dissemination in HIV patients.

B. *Diagnosis*
   - Varicella and herpes zoster are typically differentiated by its appearance and area of distribution and are regularly diagnosed clinically. Swabs of vesicular fluid from a fresh lesion or tissue biopsies taken for viral culture, direct fluorescent antigen testing, or polymerase chain reaction (PCR).

C. *Prevention*
   - Household contacts of HIV people without indication of immunity to VZV should be vaccinated to prevent varicella infection and transmission of wild-type VZV to susceptible contacts with HIV (BIII). Vaccination to Prevent Primary Infection (Varicella) The live attenuated varicella vaccine (Varivax®) proved to be harmless and immunogenic in HIV who have lesser and conserved immune systems.

D. *Treatment*
   - Antiviral therapy should be started as soon as possible for all people with HIV with herpes zoster diagnosed within 5-7days of rash onset.

# 6. Opportunistic Infections in Post-Transplants (Organ or Bone Marrow)

Opportunistic infections typically occur in less than a year of transplants in spite of following the HLA matching, cross match, and irradiating the donor blood. Human blood group system is so immunogenic that even a tiny amount of disparity is detected by our immune cells and initiate defense mechanisms against them. Recent advances made in the molecular era has shown the various immunological and various expression in the blood group system and the immunology receptor expression by the solid organs in the host. Stem cell transplant is a trend in this molecular era which a boon in treating all hematological malignancy and immunodeficiency diseases. This would give life to many young individuals with genetic diseases.

Prompt and timely use of immunosuppressants prevents transplant rejection but as a consequence it puts the host at risk of many dangerous OIs. Post transplants individuals are at higher to common infections but increased in frequency of many folds than the general population. OIs in transplant patients has to be suspected when patient with unusually severe infections caused by common pathogens (Riccardi et al., 2019b), as these pathogens take advantage of a host with a compromised immune system and/or with an altered microbiota (Riccardi et al., 2019b; Rosa et al., 2015). OIs can present as widely in the whole world as some ubiquitous organisms indwelling in the open environment, usually staying on the host as commensals. Exposures to different vast environmental factors, intrinsic virulence factors, the host at risk, especially for mycobacteria, fungi, and parasites (Bottieau, 2014; Nucci et al., 2010). These provide the ambient environment to Favour their growth and survival. Moreover, genetic host patterns and the diverse type, grade, and timing of iatrogenic immune suppression can affect both the likelihood and clinical features of OIs (De Rodriguez et al., 1994; Polvi et al., 2015).

Prevention is one of the major ways of saving the host from getting an opportunistic infection. This can be achieved by proper monitoring and starting prophylactic medication according to the immune status of the host. Nowadays lot of perfection in matching the organs and blood has evolved through many nanotechnologies which would greatly reduce the rejection. These techniques also detect early symptoms and signs of OI are which would help to initiate prompt treating the risky individuals.

## Conclusion

OIs are diseases that get awakened in a weekend immune system. Having a thorough knowledge of these diseases would help to suspect at the earliest, timely investigate and diagnose. This would help in treatment and well as prevention. Primary disease treatment and keeping them under control is the major responsibility of every patient and medical expert. Regular monitoring, counselling about the need to be on treatment and to inform if any symptoms would do the best way to prevent the OIs. High-risk individuals and patients who cannot be monitored should be started on appropriate prophylaxis Early detection, intervention, and following the appropriate regimen.

# References

Alberts, B., Johnson, A., Lewis, J. et al. (2002). B Cells and Antibodies - Molecular Biology of the Cell. In *Molecular Biology of the Cell*. New York: Garland Science. Retrieved April 26, 2022, from https://www.ncbi.nlm.nih.gov/books/NBK26884/.

Alberts, B., Johnson, A., Lewis, J., et al. (2002). Chapter 24: The Adaptive Immune System. In *Molecular Biology of the Cell*. New York: Garland Science. Retrieved April 26, 2022, from https://www.ncbi.nlm.nih.gov/books/NBK21070/.

Artal, R., Agreda, B., Serrano, E., Alfonso, J. I., & Vallés, H. (2010). Rhinocerebral mucormycosis: report on eight cases. *Acta Otorrinolaringologica Espanola*, 61(4), 301–305. https://doi.org/10.1016/j.otorri.2010.01.003.

Atkins, R. C., & Zimmet, P. (2010). Diabetic kidney disease: act now or pay later. *Saudi Journal of Kidney Diseases and Transplantation : An Official Publication of the Saudi Center for Organ Transplantation, Saudi Arabia*, 21(2), 217–221.

Bacchetti, P., Osmond, D., Chaisson, R. E., Dritz, S., Rutherford, G. W., Swig, L., & Moss, A. R. (1988). Survival patterns of the first 500 patients with AIDS in San Francisco. *The Journal of Infectious Diseases*, 157(5), 1044–1047. https://doi.org/10.1093/infdis/157.5.1044.

Bate, S. L., Dollard, S. C., & Cannon, M. J. (2010). Cytomegalovirus seroprevalence in the United States: the national health and nutrition examination surveys, 1988-2004. *Clinical Infectious Diseases: An Official Publication of the Infectious Diseases Society of America*, 50(11), 1439–1447. https://doi.org/10.1086/652438.

Bennett, J.E., Dolin, R., & Blaser, M.J. (2020). *Mandell, Douglas, and Bennett's Principles and Practice of Infectious Diseases, 9th Edition*. Elsevier. Retrieved April 24, 2022, from https://www.us.elsevierhealth.com/mandell-douglas-and-bennetts-principles-and-practice-of-infectious-diseases-9780323482554.html.

Bonacini, M., Young, T., medicine, L. L. A. of internal, & 1991, undefined. (n.d.). The causes of esophageal symptoms in human immunodeficiency virus infection: a prospective study of 110 patients. *Jamanetwork.Com*. Retrieved April 24, 2022, from https://jamanetwork.com/journals/jamainternalmedicine/article-abstract/615385.

Bottieau, E. (2014). Tropical parasitic diseases and immunosuppression. *Clinical Microbiology and Infection*, 20(4), 277. https://doi.org/10.1111/1469-0691.12590.

Calvet, H. M., & Yoshikawa, T. T. (2001). Infections in diabetes. *Infectious Disease Clinics of North America*, 15(2), 407--21, viii. https://doi.org/10.1016/s0891-5520(05)70153-7.

Carfrae, M. J., & Kesser, B. W. (2008). Malignant Otitis Externa. *Otolaryngologic Clinics of North America, 41*(3), 537–549. https://doi.org/10.1016/J.OTC.2008.01.004.

Casqueiro, J., Casqueiro, J., & Alves, C. (2012). Infections in patients with diabetes mellitus: A review of pathogenesis. *Indian Journal of Endocrinology and Metabolism, 16* (Suppl1), S27. https://doi.org/10.4103/2230-8210.94253.

Clementi, N., Ghosh, S., De Santis, M., Castelli, M., Criscuolo, E., Zanoni, I., Clementi, M., & Mancini, N. (2021). Viral Respiratory Pathogens and Lung Injury. *Clinical Microbiology Reviews, 34*(3). https://doi.org/10.1128/CMR.00103-20.

Cooper, A. M. (2009). Cell mediated immune responses in Tuberculosis. *Annual Review of Immunology, 27*, 393. https://doi.org/10.1146/ANNUREV.IMMUNOL.021908.1327 03

Cornely, O. A., Alastruey-Izquierdo, A., Arenz, D., Chen, S. C. A., Dannaoui, E., Hochhegger, B., Hoenigl, M., Jensen, H. E., Lagrou, K., Lewis, R. E., Mellinghoff, S. C., Mer, M., Pana, Z. D., Seidel, D., Sheppard, D. C., Wahba, R., Akova, M., Alanio, A., Al-Hatmi, A. M. S., Chakrabarti, A. (2019). Global guideline for the diagnosis and management of mucormycosis: an initiative of the European Confederation of Medical Mycology in cooperation with the Mycoses Study Group Education and Research Consortium. *The Lancet. Infectious Diseases, 19*(12), e405--e421. https://doi.org/10.1016/S1473-3099(19)30312-3.

Dean, N. (2021). HIV info and Clinical Info. *Medical Reference Services Quarterly, 40*(4), 421–427. https://doi.org/10.1080/02763869.2021.1987807.

DeRodriguez, C., Fuhrer, J., & Lake-Bakaar, G. (1994). Cytomegalovirus colitis in patients with acquired immunodeficiency syndrome. *Journal of the Royal Society of Medicine, 87*, 203–205.

Dybul, M., Fauci, A. S., Bartlett, J. G., Kaplan, J. E., & Pau, A. K. (2002). Guidelines for using antiretroviral agents among HIV-infected adults and adolescents: The panel on clinical practices for treatment of HIV. *Annals of Internal Medicine, 137*(5 II), 381–433. https://doi.org/10.7326/0003-4819-137-5_part_2-200209031-00001.

Geerlings, S. E., & Hoepelman, A. I. (1999). Immune dysfunction in patients with diabetes mellitus (DM). *FEMS Immunology and Medical Microbiology, 26*(3–4), 259–265. https://doi.org/10.1111/j.1574-695X.1999.tb01397.x.

Giuliani, A., Mettimano, M., Viviani, D., Scagliusi, A., Bruno, A., Russo, A., Rotoli, M., & Savi, L. (2010). An uncommon case of systemic Mucormycosis associated with spinal cord infarction in a recently diagnosed diabetic. *International Journal of Immunopathology and Pharmacology, 23*(1), 355–358. https://doi.org/10.1177/039 463201002300135.

Jabs, D. A., Van Natta, M. L., Kempen, J. H., Pavan, P. R., Lim, J. I., Murphy, R. L., & Hubbard, L. D. (2002). Characteristics of patients with cytomegalovirus retinitis in the era of highly active antiretroviral therapy. *American Journal of Ophthalmology, 133*(1), 48–61. https://doi.org/10.1016/S0002-9394(01)01322-8.

Joshi, N., Caputo, G. M., Weitekamp, M. R., & Karchmer, A. W. (1999). Infections in patients with diabetes mellitus. *The New England Journal of Medicine, 341*(25), 1906–1912. https://doi.org/10.1056/NEJM199912163412507.

Klein, R. S., Harris, C. A., Small, C. B., Moll, B., Lesser, M., & Friedland, G. H. (1984). Oral Candidiasis in High-Risk Patients as the Initial Manifestation of the Acquired

Immunodeficiency Syndrome. *New England Journal of Medicine*, *311*(6), 354–358. https://doi.org/10.1056/NEJM198408093110602.

Liu, M., Spellberg, B., Phan, Q. T., Fu, Y., Fu, Y., Lee, A. S., Edwards, J. E. J., Filler, S. G., & Ibrahim, A. S. (2010). The endothelial cell receptor GRP78 is required for mucormycosis pathogenesis in diabetic mice. *The Journal of Clinical Investigation*, *120*(6), 1914–1924. https://doi.org/10.1172/JCI42164.

Magliocca, K. R., Vivas, E. X., & Griffith, C. C. (2018). Idiopathic, Infectious and Reactive Lesions of the Ear and Temporal Bone. *Head and Neck Pathology*, *12*(3), 328–349. https://doi.org/10.1007/s12105-018-0952-0.

Marcotte, H., & Hammarström, L. (2015). Passive Immunization: Toward Magic Bullets. *Mucosal Immunology*, *2-2*, 1403. https://doi.org/10.1016/B978-0-12-415847-4.00071-9.

Muller, L. M. A. J., Gorter, K. J., Hak, E., Goudzwaard, W. L., Schellevis, F. G., Hoepelman, A. I. M., & Rutten, G. E. H. M. (2005). Increased risk of common infections in patients with type 1 and type 2 diabetes mellitus. *Clinical Infectious Diseases: An Official Publication of the Infectious Diseases Society of America*, *41*(3), 281–288. https://doi.org/10.1086/431587.

Nagasawa, T., Noda, M., Katagiri, S., Takaichi, M., Takahashi, Y., Wara-Aswapati, N., Kobayashi, H., Ohara, S., Kawaguchi, Y., Tagami, T., Furuichi, Y., & Izumi, Y. (2010). Relationship between periodontitis and diabetes - importance of a clinical study to prove the vicious cycle. *Internal Medicine (Tokyo, Japan)*, *49*(10), 881–885. https://doi.org/10.2169/internalmedicine.49.3351.

Nahid, P., Dorman, S. E., Alipanah, N., Barry, P. M., Brozek, J. L., Cattamanchi, A., Chaisson, L. H., Chaisson, R. E., Daley, C. L., Grzemska, M., Higashi, J. M., Ho, C. S., Hopewell, P. C., Keshavjee, S. A., Lienhardt, C., Menzies, R., Merrifield, C., Narita, M., O'Brien, R., Vernon, A. (2016). Official American Thoracic Society/Centers for Disease Control and Prevention/Infectious Diseases Society of America Clinical Practice Guidelines: Treatment of Drug-Susceptible Tuberculosis. *Clinical Infectious Diseases*, *63*(7), e147–e195. https://doi.org/10.1093/CID/CIW376.

Nicholson, L. B. (2016). The immune system. *Essays in Biochemistry*, *60*(3), 275. https://doi.org/10.1042/EBC20160017.

Niewiesk, S. (2014). Maternal Antibodies: Clinical Significance, Mechanism of Interference with Immune Responses, and Possible Vaccination Strategies. *Frontiers in Immunology*, *5*(SEP). https://doi.org/10.3389/FIMMU.2014.00446.

Nucci, M., Queiroz-Telles, F., Tobón, A. M., Restrepo, A., & Colombo, A. L. (2010). Epidemiology of opportunistic fungal infections in latin America. *Clinical Infectious Diseases*, *51*(5), 561–570. https://doi.org/10.1086/655683/2/51-5-561-FIG003.GIF.

O'Driscoll, B. R., Howard, L. S., & Davison, A. G. (2008). BTS guideline for emergency oxygen use in adult patients. *Thorax*, *63*(Suppl 6), vi1–vi68. https://doi.org/10.1136/THX.2008.102947.

Peleg, A. Y., Weerarathna, T., McCarthy, J. S., & Davis, T. M. E. (2007). Common infections in diabetes: pathogenesis, management and relationship to glycaemic control. *Diabetes/Metabolism Research and Reviews*, *23*(1), 3–13. https://doi.org/10.1002/dmrr.682.

Polvi, E. J., Li, X., O'Meara, T. R., Leach, M. D., & Cowen, L. E. (2015). Opportunistic yeast pathogens: reservoirs, virulence mechanisms, and therapeutic strategies. *Cellular and Molecular Life Sciences : CMLS, 72*(12), 2261–2287. https://doi.org/10.1007/S00018-015-1860-Z.

Powderly, W. G. (2010). Opportunistic infections. *Infectious Diseases: Third Edition, 2,* 964–974. https://doi.org/10.1016/B978-0-323-04579-7.00091-5.

Riccardi, N., Rotulo, G. A., & Castagnola, E. (2019a). Definition of Opportunistic Infections in Immunocompromised Children on the Basis of Etiologies and Clinical Features: A Summary for Practical Purposes. *Current Pediatric Reviews, 15*(4), 197. https://doi.org/10.2174/1573396315666190617151745.

Riccardi, N., Rotulo, G. A., & Castagnola, E. (2019b). Definition of Opportunistic Infections in Immunocompromised Children on the Basis of Etiologies and Clinical Features: A Summary for Practical Purposes. *Current Pediatric Reviews, 15*(4), 197–206. https://doi.org/10.2174/1573396315666190617151745.

Rosa, F. De, Corcione, S., Raviolo, S., Med, C. M.-I., & 2015, undefined. (2015). Candidemia, and infections by Clostridium difficile and carbapenemase-producing Enterobacteriaceae: new enteropathogenetic opportunistic syndromes. *Infezmed.It, 2,* 105–116. https://www.infezmed.it/media/journal/Vol_23_2_2015_2.pdf.

Rubin, J., & Yu, V. L. (1988). Malignant external otitis: Insights into pathogenesis, clinical manifestations, diagnosis, and therapy. *The American Journal of Medicine, 85*(3), 391–398. https://doi.org/10.1016/0002-9343(88)90592-X.

Severo, C. B., Guazzelli, L. S., & Severo, L. C. (2010). Chapter 7: Zygomycosis. *Jornal Brasileiro de Pneumologia : Publicacao Oficial Da Sociedade Brasileira de Pneumologia e Tisilogia, 36*(1), 134–141. https://doi.org/10.1590/s1806-37132010000100018.

Shanson, D. C. (1989). *Microbiology in Clinical Practice.* 657. Butterworth-Heinemann.

Skiada, A., Pavleas, I., & Drogari-Apiranthitou, M. (2020). Epidemiology and Diagnosis of Mucormycosis: An Update. *Journal of Fungi (Basel, Switzerland), 6*(4). https://doi.org/10.3390/jof6040265.

Smith, N. C., Rise, M. L., & Christian, S. L. (2019). A Comparison of the Innate and Adaptive Immune Systems in Cartilaginous Fish, Ray-Finned Fish, and Lobe-Finned Fish. *Frontiers in Immunology, 10,* 2292. https://doi.org/10.3389/FIMMU.2019.02292/BIBTEX.

Sonnenberg, P., Glynn, J. R., Fielding, K., Murray, J., Godfrey-Fausselt, P., & Shearer, S. (2005a). How soon after infection with HIV does the risk of tuberculosis start to increase? A retrospective cohort study in South African gold miners. *The Journal of Infectious Diseases, 191*(2), 150–158. https://doi.org/10.1086/426827.

Sonnenberg, P., Glynn, J. R., Fielding, K., Murray, J., Godfrey-Fausselt, P., & Shearer, S. (2005b). How soon after infection with HIV does the risk of tuberculosis start to increase? A retrospective cohort study in South African gold miners. *The Journal of Infectious Diseases, 191*(2), 150–158. https://doi.org/10.1086/426827.

Sun, J., Wang, L., Yang, C., & Song, L. (2020). An Ancient BCR-like Signaling Promotes ICP Production and Hemocyte Phagocytosis in Oyster. *IScience, 23*(2). https://doi.org/10.1016/J.ISCI.2020.100834.

Tellier, R., Li, Y., Cowling, B. J., & Tang, J. W. (2019). Recognition of aerosol transmission of infectious agents: A commentary. *BMC Infectious Diseases*, *19*(1), 1–9. https://doi.org/10.1186/S12879-019-3707-Y/FIGURES/1.

Veenstra, J., Van Praag, R. M. E., Krol, A., Wertheim Van Dillen, P. M. E., Weigel, H. M., Schellekens, P. T. A., Lange, J. M. A., Coutinho, R. A., & Van Der Meer, J. T. M. (1996). Complications of varicella zoster virus reactivation in HIV-infected homosexual men. *AIDS (London, England)*, *10*(4), 393–399. https://doi.org/10.1097/00002030-199604000-00007.

Wood, R., Maartens, G., immune, C. L.-J. of acquired, & 2000, undefined. (n.d.). Risk factors for developing tuberculosis in HIV-1-infected adults from communities with a low or very high incidence of tuberculosis. *Europepmc.Org*. Retrieved April 24, 2022, from https://europepmc.org/article/med/10708059.

World Health Organization. (2021). *Global Tuberculosis Report*. https://www.who.int/publications/i/item/9789240037021.

# Editors' Contact Information

### *Dr. Jayapradha Ramakrishnan*
Associate Professor
Centre for Research in Infectious Diseases (CRID)
School of Chemical and Biotechnology
SASTRA Deemed to be University
Thanjavur, Tamil Nadu, India
antibioticbiology@gmail.com

### *Dr. Ganesh Babu Malli Mohan*
Assistant Professor
Department of Biotechnology
School of Chemical and Biotechnology
SASTRA Deemed to be University
Thanjavur, Tamil Nadu, India
mmganeshbabumku@gmail.com

# Index

## A

*Acinetobacter baumannii* (*A. baumannii*), 108, 110, 118, 119, 120, 121
acquired immunity, 123, 127, 128, 129, 130
acquired immunodeficiency syndrome, 137, 147
adaptive immunity, 75, 104, 113, 127, 128
AIDS, vii, 5, 20, 28, 29, 31, 34, 77, 93, 98, 124, 137, 138, 141, 146, 150
alveolar macrophage, 6, 21, 78
antibiotic resistance, 116, 118, 119
antibiotics, 3, 87, 105, 106, 107, 108, 109, 110, 112, 113, 120, 121, 131
antibodies, 73, 74, 76, 78, 82, 83, 84, 86, 87, 88, 91, 92, 95, 97, 98, 99, 100, 103, 127, 128, 129, 146, 148
antifungal, 11, 17, 18, 28, 30, 32, 38, 72, 73, 78, 79, 80, 94, 95, 96, 97, 100, 101, 103, 104, 131
antigen, 27, 30, 35, 75, 76, 77, 81, 85, 89, 91, 93, 94, 127, 128, 142, 144
antimicrobial resistance, vii, 11, 105, 107, 109, 117, 119, 120
antiviral agents, 72
ART, 20, 124, 137, 139, 141, 143
aspergillosis, 38, 72, 75, 81, 95, 98, 99, 100, 101, 102, 103, 104

## B

bacteremia, 108, 109, 110, 119

bacteria, vii, 43, 71, 73, 77, 84, 85, 86, 94, 106, 107, 108, 113, 114, 115, 116, 119, 121, 123, 124, 135, 139, 141
bacterial infection, 72, 81, 84, 87, 100, 103, 105, 106, 107, 111, 125, 142
bacterial pneumonia, vii
Bacteriophage Recombineering of Electroporated DNA (BRED), 114, 119, 120
bacteriophages, v, viii, 105, 106, 107, 108, 109, 110, 111, 112, 113, 116, 117, 118, 119, 120
biopsy, 17, 144
blood, 1, 8, 11, 81, 91, 99, 102, 111, 125, 127, 132, 134, 137, 138, 139, 142, 145
bone, 11, 17, 19, 26, 29, 120, 123, 125, 130
brain, 3, 4, 7, 16, 19, 25, 27, 133, 138

## C

cancer, vii, 3, 11, 20, 72, 73, 76, 78, 82, 83, 86, 89, 94, 96, 100, 101, 102, 123, 125, 130, 133, 138
candidiasis, vii, 38, 72, 81, 95, 98, 100, 104, 142
CD8+, 74, 86, 87, 92, 93, 98, 103
cell death, 22, 33, 76, 85, 134
central nervous system (CNS), 133, 138, 140, 144
chemotherapy, 20, 32, 98, 100, 101, 119, 121, 130, 134
chimeric antigen receptor (CAR), 8, 77, 91, 92, 94, 99, 102

chimeric antigen receptor T-cells (CAR-T), 77, 91
ChIP (chromatin immunoprecipitation), 9
clinical presentation, 11, 124, 140, 143
clinical trials, 83, 84, 85, 87, 91, 92, 102, 116
contaminated food, 44, 125, 141
corticosteroid therapy, 14, 20, 141
corticosteroids, 6, 14, 33, 77, 79
COVID-19, vii, 13, 14, 30, 37, 44, 47, 54, 55, 58, 59, 63, 64, 65, 66, 67, 70, 125, 135, 136
cranial nerve, 15, 16, 133
CRISPR, 106, 113, 114, 115, 116, 117, 118, 119
CRISPR-Cas-Mediated Genome Engineering, 115
cryptococcal meningitis, vii, 20, 30, 31, 37, 38, 98, 138
cryptococcosis, 1, 18, 20, 25, 26, 31, 34, 35, 36, 37, 72, 80, 97
Cryptococcus neoformans (*C. neoformans*), 18, 19, 20, 21, 22, 23, 24, 25, 27, 30, 32, 33, 34, 35, 36, 37, 39, 81, 97, 101
*Cryptococcus* spp., 1, 19, 24, 25, 27
CSF, 30, 75, 78, 79, 87, 93, 94, 102
culture, 16, 26, 27, 89, 140, 141, 142, 143, 144
Cutaneous (Skin) Mucormycosis, 12, 15, 36
cystic fibrosis, 74, 96, 111
cytokine, 72, 74, 75, 77, 78, 80, 81, 82, 83, 85, 87, 88, 89, 90, 91, 92, 93, 94, 101, 104, 135, 136
cytomegalovirus, 94, 95, 147
cytotoxicity, 76, 84, 101

## D

deaths, 77, 105, 109, 132, 139
defense mechanisms, 38, 79, 124, 145
deficiency, 123, 130, 131
degradation, 23, 113, 117

dendritic cell (DC), 79, 81, 83, 87, 88, 90, 93, 95, 98, 101, 102, 127
dengue, 57, 63, 68, 69
detection, 27, 30, 34, 104, 140, 142, 146
diabetes, 3, 6, 11, 12, 14, 30, 31, 37, 38, 123, 124, 125, 131, 133, 135, 136, 142, 146, 147, 148
Diabetes Mellitus (DM), 6, 12, 14, 30, 35, 123, 125, 131, 132, 133, 134, 147
diabetic ketoacidosis, 6, 7, 11, 31, 132
diagnostics, 1, 34, 140
diarrhea, 74, 75, 110, 142
diseases, vii, 1, 9, 12, 13, 14, 20, 31, 32, 33, 34, 35, 36, 37, 41, 42, 43, 46, 51, 52, 59, 60, 61, 63, 64, 68, 69, 70, 72, 76, 78, 82, 86, 90, 94, 95, 96, 98, 99, 100, 101, 102, 103, 104, 110, 117, 121, 122, 124, 125, 131, 135, 138, 145, 146
disseminated mucormycosis, 4, 12, 16
DNA, 24, 88, 93, 97, 107, 113, 114, 116
drugs, 6, 8, 31, 71, 72, 73, 78, 83, 85, 97, 100, 104, 108, 110, 123, 130, 135

## E

Ebola Virus Disease (EVD), 42, 43, 56, 62, 63, 64, 65, 68, 69
emergence, 1, 32, 48, 54, 55, 58, 71, 106, 110, 116, 120
encoding, 10, 98, 102, 107
engineering, viii, 91, 97, 106, 113, 114, 115, 117, 118, 119, 120
*Enterococcus faecium*is (*E. faecium*), 108
environment, 2, 8, 10, 19, 20, 21, 24, 43, 44, 46, 68, 106, 123, 132, 134, 142, 145
enzyme, 7, 22, 23, 27, 73, 107, 109, 110, 127, 130
epidemic spreading, 41, 61, 66
epidemics, vii, 41, 42, 43, 44, 46, 47, 51, 52, 53, 54, 55, 56, 57, 58, 59, 60, 61, 62, 63, 64, 65, 66, 67, 68, 69, 70
epidemiology, 1, 11, 12, 20, 34, 37, 38, 43, 57, 62, 64, 65, 68, 96, 98, 100, 120, 148, 149

epidermal growth factor receptor (EFGR), 11
epithelial cells, 5, 96, 134
epitopes, 87, 99, 104
ESKAPE pathogens, 106, 108, 112, 117, 120
evolution, 1, 33, 56, 118, 121
exposure, 5, 44, 127, 128, 140, 142

## F

fever, 25, 26, 43, 68, 69, 70, 137, 140, 142, 144
fibrosis, 74, 96, 111
fluid, 25, 55, 96, 144
food, 10, 44, 109, 118, 125, 139, 141
fungal disease, 1, 13, 72, 95, 101, 104
fungal infection, vii, 1, 2, 13, 14, 18, 30, 34, 36, 73, 77, 78, 79, 80, 82, 83, 95, 96, 98, 100, 101, 102, 104, 135, 136, 148
fungi, 2, 5, 7, 8, 9, 18, 19, 22, 24, 31, 32, 33, 34, 36, 38, 43, 71, 73, 77, 78, 79, 81, 83, 94, 98, 101, 104, 123, 124, 125, 131, 133, 134, 135, 145, 149

## G

gastrointestinal mucormycosis (GIMucormycosis), 3, 12, 15, 38
gastrointestinal tract, 73, 108, 134, 138
genes, 6, 7, 8, 9, 10, 11, 22, 23, 24, 31, 32, 33, 35, 36, 38, 91, 93, 102, 107, 112, 114, 115, 116, 130
genetic engineering, viii, 113, 117
genome, 8, 9, 10, 11, 36, 37, 106, 107, 112, 113, 114, 115, 116, 118, 119, 120, 121
genome rebooting, 114
glucose, 14, 24, 134
granulocyte transfusion (GTX), 81, 95, 104
growth, 6, 7, 8, 9, 10, 18, 23, 75, 76, 78, 94, 103, 111, 116, 119, 127, 145

## H

health, 42, 45, 46, 47, 58, 59, 70, 77, 94, 101, 105, 108, 109, 118, 120, 121, 132, 141, 146
*Helicobacter pylori*, 96, 97, 102
herpes, vii, 99, 131, 138, 143, 144
histoplasmosis, 72, 138
HIV-1, 92, 100, 102, 150
homologous recombination (HR), 113, 115, 116, 120
hospital, 14, 108, 110, 118, 120, 121, 125
host, vii, 1, 5, 6, 7, 8, 10, 11, 12, 22, 25, 43, 44, 52, 58, 67, 73, 76, 78, 79, 80, 82, 83, 84, 89, 90, 93, 94, 95, 96, 98, 99, 100, 102, 106, 112, 113, 114, 115, 116, 118, 119, 121, 123, 124, 127, 128, 134, 135, 137, 138, 139, 145
host defense, 1, 7, 90, 99, 118, 124
host pathogen interactions, vii, 52
human, 2, 6, 22, 24, 32, 37, 44, 53, 54, 55, 57, 63, 64, 67, 68, 74, 77, 79, 84, 86, 87, 89, 91, 92, 94, 95, 96, 97, 99, 102, 103, 105, 108, 109, 123, 133, 146
Human Immunodeficiency Virus (HIV), vii, 12, 21, 28, 31, 35, 37, 77, 85, 91, 92, 93, 96, 97, 98, 99, 100, 102, 123, 124, 125, 130, 131, 137, 138, 139, 140, 141, 142, 143, 144, 147, 149, 150
humoral immunity, 82, 88, 127, 132
hyperglycemia, 6, 14, 32, 132
hypoxia, 15, 18, 135

## I

IFN, 74, 75, 85, 86, 87, 88, 89, 90, 93, 98, 103
IFNγ, 79, 80
immune response, 22, 44, 73, 74, 79, 83, 85, 87, 88, 89, 93, 98, 100, 101, 102, 127, 128, 130, 135, 138, 147
immune system, vii, 3, 44, 71, 72, 73, 76, 78, 81, 83, 85, 86, 87, 96, 100, 115, 123, 124, 125, 126, 127, 128, 130, 131, 137, 138, 144, 145, 148

# Index

immunity, vii, 32, 42, 48, 49, 50, 51, 55, 59, 61, 64, 67, 68, 69, 72, 75, 76, 77, 78, 80, 81, 82, 83, 87, 88, 89, 90, 91, 94, 95, 96, 97, 99, 100, 101, 102, 104, 113, 123, 124, 125, 126, 127, 128, 129, 130, 132, 135, 137, 139, 144
immunization, 64, 76, 93, 132
immunocompromised, vii, 2, 4, 6, 19, 72, 77, 123, 149
immunodeficiency, 77, 99, 124, 130, 131, 135, 137, 139, 140, 145, 146, 147
immunoglobulins, 74, 76, 82, 86, 95, 128, 129
immunological memory, 73, 76, 128, 129
immunomodulation, v, viii, 71, 73, 74, 77, 84, 90, 94, 96, 97, 98
immunomodulatory, 72, 78, 88, 89, 102
immunosuppression, 1, 6, 20, 101, 142, 143, 146
immunotherapy, v, viii, 71, 72, 73, 74, 75, 76, 77, 82, 83, 87, 88, 89, 90, 91, 92, 93, 94, 95, 96, 97, 98, 99, 100, 101, 102
in vitro, 6, 92, 110, 114, 116, 119
in vivo, 32, 99, 107, 110, 113, 116
India, viii, 1, 3, 11, 12, 13, 14, 20, 32, 37, 41, 66, 67, 105, 123, 151
infections, v, vii, 1, 2, 3, 4, 5, 6, 11, 12, 13, 18, 19, 20, 24, 25, 26, 28, 30, 31, 32, 34, 35, 36, 38, 42, 44, 45, 46, 47, 49, 50, 52, 54, 55, 57, 62, 63, 64, 65, 67, 68, 69, 70, 71, 72, 73, 74, 75, 76, 77, 78, 79, 80, 81, 82, 83, 84, 85, 86, 87, 88, 89, 90, 91, 92, 93, 94, 95, 96, 97, 98, 99, 100, 101, 102, 103, 104, 105, 106, 107, 108, 109, 110, 111, 112, 117, 118, 119, 120, 121, 122, 123, 124, 125, 127, 128, 129, 130, 131, 132, 133, 134, 135, 136, 137, 138, 139, 140, 141, 142, 143, 144, 145, 146, 147, 148, 149
infectious disease, vii, 35, 41, 42, 44, 46, 51, 52, 59, 60, 61, 62, 64, 65, 67, 69, 86, 90, 98, 99, 100, 102, 104, 117
inflammation, 77, 85, 96, 99, 104
influenza, 42, 43, 45, 47, 52, 54, 55, 56, 60, 61, 62, 63, 64, 65, 68, 69, 91, 97
injuries, 11, 15, 17, 96, 103, 123, 134
innate immunity, 72, 82, 90, 91, 126
interferon, 75, 97, 101, 103, 127
interferon-γ, 75, 97, 101
intravenously, 80
iron, 6, 7, 10, 14, 31, 33, 34, 38

## K

Kaposi sarcoma, 73, 90, 138
ketoacidosis, 6, 7, 11, 31, 32, 132
kidney, 2, 3, 11, 12, 17, 19, 146
killer cells, 22, 82, 86, 101, 103
*Klebsiella pneumoniae* (*K. pneumoniae*), 84, 108, 110, 117, 121, 122

## L

lead, vii, 15, 25, 85, 93, 124, 134
lesions, 15, 25, 29, 86, 91, 141, 142
ligand, 76, 86, 95, 97, 102
liver, 7, 19, 20, 103, 108
lymphocytes, 22, 74, 76, 85, 86, 88, 127
lymphoid, 85, 88, 101
lysis, 92, 107, 113, 115

## M

mAb, 72, 83, 84
macrophages, 6, 22, 76, 78, 79, 84, 87, 89, 90, 94, 101, 127
major histocompatibility complex (MHC), 82, 85, 87, 91, 93, 104
malaria, 67, 77, 88, 97, 102
management, 32, 33, 36, 38, 53, 58, 67, 102, 104, 121, 125, 133, 141, 143, 147, 148
marrow, 11, 103, 123, 125, 130
mathematical modeling, vii, 41, 42, 46, 58, 63, 67, 70
medical, vii, 31, 56, 94, 95, 101, 106, 107, 109, 116, 120, 123, 125, 132, 133, 136, 137, 146
medication, vii, 3, 17, 90, 133, 135, 136, 145

medicine, 17, 34, 36, 37, 52, 62, 64, 67, 95, 97, 99, 100, 119, 121, 136, 146
mellitus, 6, 12, 14, 30, 131, 133, 135, 147, 148
memory, 73, 76, 93, 127, 128, 129
meningitis, vii, 20, 28, 30, 31, 37, 38, 98, 108, 110, 138, 140, 141
meta-analysis, 34, 61, 121
metabolism, 7, 10, 130
mice, 80, 81, 84, 86, 88, 89, 90, 95, 96, 97, 100, 102, 103, 148
microbes, vii, 32, 61, 71, 72, 73, 76, 78, 79, 81, 84, 88, 89, 90, 94, 95, 101, 102, 103, 118, 119, 121
microorganisms, 85, 94, 123, 124, 127
modelling, 51, 52, 53, 54, 55, 57, 58, 60, 61, 62, 65
models, 41, 42, 44, 45, 46, 47, 48, 51, 52, 53, 54, 55, 56, 57, 58, 59, 60, 61, 62, 63, 64, 65, 66, 68, 69, 79, 81, 84, 86, 91, 92, 97, 109
molecules, 76, 82, 85, 127
monoclonal antibodies (mAbs), 71, 72, 74, 76, 83, 84, 88, 89
monocyte-derived macrophages (MDMs), 22, 84
morbidity, 1, 30, 43, 58, 72, 125, 132, 133, 138, 139
mortality, 1, 2, 6, 14, 20, 30, 31, 43, 48, 58, 59, 72, 80, 97, 103, 125, 133, 136, 138, 139
mRNA, 11, 93, 98
*Mucor* spp., 1, 2
mucoralean fungi, 5
mucormycosis, 1, 2, 3, 4, 5, 6, 7, 9, 11, 12, 13, 14, 15, 16, 17, 18, 31, 32, 33, 34, 35, 36, 37, 38, 39, 131, 132, 133, 134, 136, 146, 147, 148, 149
mucormycosis pathogenesis, 6, 148
mutation, 56, 113, 114, 115, 116, 123, 130, 136, 138
mycology, 31, 33, 35, 36, 37, 99, 101

**N**

natural killer (NK), 22, 76, 82, 85, 86, 89, 93, 101, 102, 103, 104
nerve, 15, 16, 133, 144
nervous system, 31, 133, 138, 140, 144
neutropenia, 2, 3, 5, 11, 12, 77, 79, 81, 125, 134
neutrophils, 5, 32, 79, 80, 86, 95, 132
NK cells, 82, 85, 86, 89, 93, 102
nodes, 25, 45, 53, 54

**O**

omics, viii, 1, 8, 9, 31
opportunistic, v, vii, 1, 14, 18, 20, 25, 30, 38, 71, 72, 73, 74, 77, 81, 83, 84, 88, 90, 94, 108, 109, 111, 118, 123, 124, 125, 132, 133, 135, 136, 137, 138, 139, 144, 145, 148, 149
opportunistic fungal infections, 1, 14, 77, 148
opportunistic infections (OIs), vii, 71, 73, 77, 79, 84, 94, 123, 124, 125, 133, 137, 138, 144, 145, 149
orbit, 18, 134, 138
organ, vii, 3, 11, 12, 13, 36, 72, 77, 123, 130, 131, 134, 138, 143
organism, 3, 6, 14, 17, 22, 24, 111, 124, 127, 128, 138, 140, 142
organs, 1, 2, 4, 7, 25, 27, 132, 139, 143, 145
osteomyelitis, 110, 133
oxygen, 8, 18, 33, 34, 135, 148

**P**

pain, 15, 16, 25, 26, 133, 134
pandemics, vii, 20, 31, 42, 43, 47, 50, 52, 55, 58, 63, 68, 135
parasites, 17, 43, 44, 69, 71, 72, 73, 77, 88, 94, 96, 97, 123, 125, 145
pathogen, v, vii, 1, 2, 6, 7, 8, 9, 18, 30, 31, 32, 34, 38, 41, 44, 45, 46, 58, 60, 72, 87, 88, 96, 97, 98, 100, 101, 105, 106, 107, 108, 109, 110, 111, 112, 116, 118, 119,

120, 123, 124, 125, 127, 128, 132, 134, 135, 145, 147, 149
pathogenesis, 10, 33, 34, 95, 96, 99, 108, 118, 119, 125, 147, 148, 149
pathway, 4, 6, 11, 22, 35, 36, 39, 83, 85, 86, 93, 94, 100, 104, 115
PCR, 16, 24, 115, 140, 142, 144
peptide, 5, 10, 82, 92, 93, 104, 107
pH, 6, 8, 10, 21, 134
phage, vii, 105, 106, 107, 108, 109, 110, 111, 112, 113, 114, 115, 116, 117, 118, 119, 120, 121
phage therapy, vii, 105, 106, 107, 108, 110, 111, 112, 113, 116, 117, 118, 119, 120
phagocytic cells, 77, 78, 79
phagocytosis, 11, 21, 74, 81, 132
Platelet-Derived Growth Factor Receptor B (PDGFRB), 5, 11
pleiotropic drug resistance (PDR), 8, 35
pneumonia, vii, 17, 25, 74, 81, 84, 101, 109, 131, 138
point mutation, 115, 116
polymicrobial infections, 112
population, 24, 42, 43, 46, 47, 48, 50, 53, 54, 56, 57, 58, 62, 63, 64, 65, 66, 124, 139, 141, 143, 144, 145
post-transplant infection, 124
pregnancy, 129, 130, 135
prevention, 35, 55, 103, 136, 145
progressive multifocal leukoencephalopathy, 73, 90
proliferation, 76, 77, 79, 86, 89, 92, 93, 98, 124
prophylactic, 123, 135, 136, 145
prophylaxis, 84, 96, 137, 138, 142, 146
protection, 76, 94, 97, 103, 104, 127, 128, 129
protective role, 80, 81, 82, 88
proteins, 8, 10, 77, 81, 82, 95, 106, 114
*Pseudomonas aeruginosa* (*P. aeruginosa*), 83, 84, 94, 96, 101, 108, 111, 117, 118, 119, 121, 122, 133
public health, 42, 47, 70, 101, 105, 109, 118
pulmonary mucormycosis, 3, 12, 15, 17, 35

# R

receptor, 5, 8, 11, 32, 75, 76, 77, 78, 86, 88, 89, 90, 91, 92, 94, 96, 97, 99, 100, 102, 111, 113, 134, 135, 145, 148
recombinant cytokines, 75, 78, 94
recombination, 113, 114, 115, 116, 120
replication, 9, 44, 91, 92, 107, 121
resistance, vii, 8, 11, 32, 36, 38, 52, 60, 65, 71, 72, 73, 78, 85, 89, 90, 94, 95, 97, 98, 99, 104, 105, 107, 108, 109, 111, 113, 116, 117, 118, 119, 120, 127, 141
response, 11, 15, 22, 32, 44, 47, 56, 73, 74, 81, 85, 88, 89, 93, 97, 98, 101, 103, 113, 118, 127, 128, 130, 132, 135, 138, 142
rhino, 13, 31, 39, 132, 138
Rhino Orbital Cerebral Mucormycosis (ROCM), 3, 12, 15, 16, 18
*Rhizopus* spp., 1, 2, 3, 7, 9, 32, 33, 38, 82, 102, 133, 134
risk, 1, 3, 5, 12, 61, 77, 83, 84, 103, 123, 125, 129, 131, 133, 136, 137, 138, 139, 140, 141, 142, 144, 145, 146, 148, 149
RNA, 9, 11, 81, 93, 107, 118
RNA sequencing, 9, 11
RNAi, 9, 10, 32, 36

# S

*Salmonella*, 63, 131, 141
SARS, 43, 61, 65
SARS-CoV, 61, 65
secondary infections, vii, 47
secretion, 73, 83, 92, 127, 131
sensitivity, 23, 44, 78, 111, 117
sepsis, 30, 95, 103, 109, 110
serum, 7, 28, 32, 104, 134
side effects, 28, 31, 90, 117
simulation, 53, 56, 58, 59, 62, 63, 66, 67
sinuses, 3, 16, 134
SIR models, 41, 47, 48, 51, 54, 55, 61
skin, 2, 4, 6, 11, 12, 19, 25, 26, 27, 29, 109, 127, 134
species, 2, 16, 19, 24, 33, 37, 44, 51, 56, 73, 82, 83, 84, 85, 90, 93, 95, 106, 108, 126, 127

stability, 11, 36, 59, 60, 61, 63, 64, 68, 70
*Staphylococcus aureus (S. aureus)*, 84, 87, 100, 108, 109, 117, 119, 121, 131
starvation, 10, 23, 34, 39
stress, 22, 23, 39, 102
structure, 8, 9, 24, 33, 46, 53, 63, 68, 69, 76
sun, 35, 62, 102, 103, 104, 127, 149
suppression, 6, 79, 92, 93, 142, 145
survival, 18, 21, 23, 30, 34, 81, 86, 93, 103, 125, 134, 145
susceptibility, 31, 38, 44, 132, 140
swelling, 9, 15, 16, 17, 21, 26, 134
symptoms, 15, 16, 25, 26, 44, 45, 128, 137, 140, 144, 145, 146
syndrome, 130, 131, 135, 136, 137, 147

## T

target, 23, 31, 73, 76, 83, 86, 94, 106, 107, 113, 115
T-cells, 14, 72, 73, 74, 75, 76, 77, 80, 82, 85, 86, 87, 89, 90, 91, 92, 93, 95, 96, 98, 99, 100, 102, 103, 127, 128, 130, 132
temperature, 10, 46, 73, 140
therapy, vii, 4, 12, 14, 18, 20, 28, 29, 30, 32, 35, 38, 71, 72, 76, 78, 79, 80, 90, 91, 92, 93, 94, 95, 96, 97, 98, 100, 101, 102, 103, 105, 106, 107, 108, 110, 111, 112, 113, 116, 117, 118, 119, 120, 121, 123, 125, 130, 131, 133, 134, 135, 137, 139, 141, 142, 143, 144, 147, 149
tissue, 14, 15, 16, 17, 18, 27, 39, 85, 134, 143, 144
TNF, 6, 75, 80, 88, 89, 99
toll-like receptors (TLRs), 5, 75, 90, 91, 96
toxicity, 31, 33, 71, 72, 116
toxoplasmosis, vii, 73, 75, 90, 97
transmission, 4, 44, 45, 47, 53, 55, 56, 57, 64, 67, 68, 69, 70, 99, 108, 138, 144, 150
transplant, vii, 3, 4, 11, 12, 13, 29, 34, 36, 38, 72, 77, 96, 100, 108, 124, 125, 130, 131, 144, 145

transplantation, 12, 79, 80, 81, 82, 95, 97, 100, 101, 103, 104, 123
treatment, v, vii, 1, 11, 17, 18, 27, 28, 30, 32, 33, 35, 36, 38, 41, 45, 56, 57, 58, 59, 65, 66, 68, 69, 70, 72, 78, 79, 80, 81, 82, 83, 84, 85, 87, 88, 89, 91, 92, 93, 95, 96, 97, 98, 100, 101, 102, 103, 105, 107, 108, 109, 110, 111, 112, 113, 116, 118, 119, 120,121, 125, 129, 130, 131, 133, 135, 138, 140, 141, 143, 144, 145, 147, 148
tuberculosis (TB), vii, 11, 51, 63, 74, 77, 83, 84, 85, 86, 87, 96, 97, 98, 99, 104, 131, 138, 139, 140, 141, 147, 148, 149, 150
tumor, 96, 100, 133

## U

uncontrolled diabetes, 11, 124, 133, 142
United States, 20, 32, 36, 58, 59, 146
upper respiratory tract, 109, 110, 135
urinary tract, 69, 74, 108, 110, 111

## V

vaccines, 44, 70, 76, 81, 93, 95, 97, 99, 101, 102, 104, 128, 132, 136, 144
viral infection, 72, 90, 91
virulence, 1, 6, 7, 8, 10, 11, 22, 24, 32, 35, 36, 37, 39, 44, 56, 73, 84, 101, 112, 118, 122, 123, 124, 132, 145, 149
virulence genes, 10, 22
viruses, 43, 56, 57, 71, 73, 77, 90, 91, 94, 105, 106, 121, 123, 125, 136

## W

water, 6, 44, 125, 137, 139, 142
white blood cells, 11, 125, 127, 137
World Health Organization (WHO), 42, 105, 108, 121, 139, 150

## Y

yeast, 18, 21, 23, 24, 27, 116, 118, 149

**Z**

Zika, 43, 57, 59, 60, 63, 70

zygomycosis, 2, 37, 72, 149